SYNOPSIS OF NEUROANATOMY

Synopsis of
Neuroanatomy

FOURTH EDITION

HOWARD A. MATZKE, Ph.D.

PROFESSOR EMERITUS
DEPARTMENT OF ANATOMY
UNIVERSITY OF KANSAS MEDICAL CENTER

FLOYD M. FOLTZ, Ph.D.

PROFESSOR
DEPARTMENT OF ANATOMY
UNIVERSITY OF KANSAS MEDICAL CENTER

NEW YORK   OXFORD
OXFORD UNIVERSITY PRESS
1983

Copyright © 1967, 1972, 1979, 1983 by Oxford University Press, Inc.

Library of Congress Cataloging in Publication Data
Matzke, Howard A.
Synopsis of neuroanatomy.
Bibliography: p.   Includes index.
. Neuroanatomy. I. Foltz, Floyd M.   II. Title.
[DNLM: 1. Nervous system—Anatomy and histology.
WL 101 M44 7s]
QM451.M32   1983   611'.8   82-13532
ISBN 0-19-503244-6 (pbk.)

Printing (last digit) : 9 8 7 6 5 4 3 2 1

Printed in the United States of America

Preface

The explosion of knowledge in neurobiology has necessitated an updating of information in this revision. To this end all chapters have been revised to varying degrees. For the sake of brevity it was necessary to be highly selective. In particular, additions or changes have been made in the following areas: neurotransmitters, Rexed's laminae, muscle spindles, pain mechanisms, organization of the retina, reticular formation, and blood-brain barrier. Two new illustrations have been added and four others revised. To make room for these changes, references to evolutionary development have been deleted.

The authors wish to express their appreciation to their many colleagues and students for valuable suggestions and criticisms: to Dr. Francisco Martinez for preparing the new and revised illustrations; to Dr. Marek Gosek for carefully reading the manuscript; to Mrs. Grace Foltz for typing the manuscript and, finally, to the staff of Oxford University Press for their patience and helpful suggestions.

Kansas City, Kansas   H.A.M.
1983   F.M.F.

Preface to the first edition

The authors undertook the writing of this book because there is a need for a clear, concise, and yet comprehensive account of neuroanatomy. Concepts are emphasized and wherever possible, evolutionary development of each system is included. It was felt this would lead to a better understanding of the organization and dynamics of the human nervous system. Clinical applications are included only where they clearly aid in the understanding of the anatomy and physiology.

The authors wish to express their appreciation to Mr. P. A. Roberts, to Mr. Alan Cole, and to Dr. Nestor Bautista, who prepared the illustrations; to Mrs. Yvonne Roberts, Mrs. Grace Foltz, Mrs. Grace Matzke, and Mrs. Annette Richberg for typing various portions of this manuscript; to their many colleagues, graduate students, and medical students for reviewing and criticizing the work; and finally, to the staff of the Oxford University Press for their patience and many helpful suggestions throughout the preparation of this book.

Kansas City, Kansas   H.A.M.
1967   F.M.F.

Contents

CONTENTS

SYNOPSIS OF NEUROANATOMY

1

Introduction

The nervous system of all but the simplest metazoans is built upon a foundation of the same basic elements. It exhibits the primary phenomena of irritability and conductivity. The nervous system first appears in coelenterates, although contractile elements which may be referred to as muscle cells are found in Porifera. The simplest element is the epithelial muscle cell (Fig. 1), which has receptive and contractile ends. The separation of these two ends results in a muscle cell and a neurosensory cell, the latter being both receptive and conductive. The final step is the formation of a true nerve cell, concerned primarily with conduction, interposed between the two previous cells. Subsequent development of the nervous system depends largely on the increase in the number and connections of these neurons.

Distinct organizational modifications first appear in archaic vertebrate ancestry, and it is here that we first see the appearance of a dorsal tubular nervous system. Afferent (sensory) fibers arising from receptors in the periphery conduct information into the central nervous system, where it is modified and integrated and then directed to the appropriate effector apparatus (muscles and glands) by way of efferent (motor) fibers. The degree to which the response is modified and delayed is directly related to the complexity of the central nervous system.

The basic subdivisions of the central nervous system are present in all vertebrates (Fig. 2); the caudal portion, i.e. the spinal

1

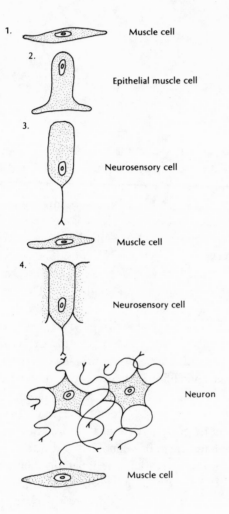

1. Muscle cell

2. Epithelial muscle cell

3. Neurosensory cell

Muscle cell

4. Neurosensory cell

Neuron

Muscle cell

1. Evolution of the Neuron

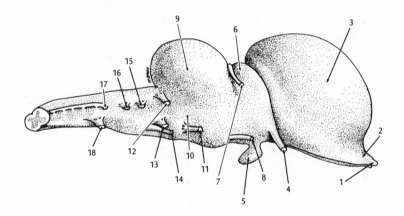

2. Generalized Vertebrate Brain and Cranial Nerves

1. I Olfactory   2. Olfactory bulb   3. Telencephalon   4. II Optic
5. Hypophysis   6. Tectum of midbrain   7. IV Trochlear   8. III
Oculomotor   9. Cerebellum   10. Rhombencephalon   11. V Trigeminal   12. VIII Auditory   13. VII Facial   14. VI Abducens
15. IX Glossopharyngeal   16. X Vagus   17. XI Spinal accessory
18. XII Hypoglossal

cord, undergoes the least amount of change in phylogeny. The cephalic portion of the primitive neural tube differentiates into three primary brain vesicles. They are, from rostal to caudal: prosencephalon, mesencephalon, and rhombencephalon. The prosencephalon further divides into the telencephalon and diencephalon, and the rhombencephalon divides into the metencephalon and myelencephalon. From these vesicles develop the various adult structures of the brain. The telencephalon is divided into two halves called cerebral hemispheres. Each half contains a cavity, the lateral ventricle, which is an enlargement of the primitive central canal. The telencephalon gives rise to the cerebral cortex and basal ganglia, and the first cranial nerve (olfactory) is attached at this level.

The diencephalon is separated into two halves by a midline third ventricle, which communicates with the lateral ventricles by way of the interventricular foramen. In the adult the diencephalon is divided into the epithalamus, dorsal thalamus, subthalamus, and hypothalamus. The second cranial nerve (optic) enters the diencephalon.

Centrally the mesencephalon contains a constricted portion of the ventricular system, the cerebral aqueduct, which communicates with the third ventricle above. The third (oculomotor) and fourth (trochlear) cranial nerves are associated with the midbrain. The tectum, containing the corpora quadrigemina (inferior and superior colliculi), is dorsal to the aqueduct, whereas the tegmentum lies ventral.

The metencephalon differentiates into the cerebellum dorsally and the pons ventrally. The fifth (trigeminal), sixth (abducens), seventh (facial), and eighth (auditory) nerves attach to the pons.

The myelencephalon develops into the medulla oblongata. The ninth (glossopharyngeal), tenth (vagus), eleventh (accessory), and twelfth (hypoglossal) cranial nerves are associated

4

with the medulla. The fourth ventricle is related to the pons and medulla ventrally, and the cerebellum dorsally. It is continuous with the cerebral aqueduct cephalically, and with the central canal, caudally.

In the lower vertebrates the spinal cord is concerned largely with basic reflex mechanisms. As the various centers in the rostral portion, i.e. brain, become progressively more important, longitudinal tracts appear. These are located at the periphery of the neuraxis. The ascending tracts carry sensory information to various parts of the brain, where it is integrated and modified. Descending motor paths from the brain can markedly modify the basic reflex mechanisms of the spinal cord; such mechanisms exist, however, even in the highest vertebrates. Differentiation and encephalization are the principal features of the phylogenetic development of the central nervous system. Formation of specific nuclear groups and fiber paths appear progressively as the nervous system becomes more complex. Concurrently there is an increase in volume and importance of the cerebral cortex and its associated thalamic nuclei. This differentiation allows for a higher degree of discrimination in sensory perception and motor activity. Older diffuse pathways, however, still persist even in man, for it is generally true that once a structure appears in phylogeny it is never lost, although the size and function of these structures may be greatly modified by phylogenetically newer portions and by the animal's specialized adaptation to its habitat.

The increase in cortex and related subcortical areas, particularly the thalamus, results in a concomitant increase in the number of interneuronal connections. The ability of the animal to modify the response to a given set of afferent stimuli and to store information (memory) is proportional to the number and complexity of these connections. The capacities to plan and show concern for the future, to develop abstract reasoning, to use language and symbols, and to demonstrate an individual personality, are probably likewise functions of a highly developed cortex and thalamus. These faculties are usually reserved for man, but no doubt the rudimentary beginnings of some of them appear in certain subhuman forms.

2

Basic Elements of the Nervous System

The nerve cell (neuron) contains a cell body (perikaryon) and processes (axon and dendrites). Neurons vary in size and shape as well as in the number of processes they possess. Unipolar neurons (Fig. 3C) have but one process, which bifurcates. Unipolar neurons are found in the sensory ganglia associated with the dorsal roots of the spinal nerves and in sensory ganglia of certain of the cranial nerves. Bipolar neurons (Fig. 3D), which have two processes, are located in the retina, olfactory membrane, and ganglia of the eighth (auditory) cranial nerve. Multipolar neurons (Fig. 3A) have three or more processes, one of which is an axon and the others dendrites, and are located in the central nervous system and autonomic ganglia. Based on the length of the axon, neurons may be designated as Golgi type I, which have long axons, or Golgi type II with short axons.

The cell body contains a prominent nucleus (Fig. 3A) (usually centrally placed) with one or more nucleoli and a light staining chromatin net. The nucleolus contains ribonucleic acid (RNA), which is also distributed throughout the nucleoplasm. The chromatin contains deoxyribonucleic acid (DNA). Scattered throughout the cytoplasm—except at the point of attachment of the axon, which is known as the axon hillock—are clumps of material called Nissl bodies (chromidial or tigroid substance). Nissl bodies, which also extend into the dendrites, vary from a fine powdery substance to regular block-like granules.

7

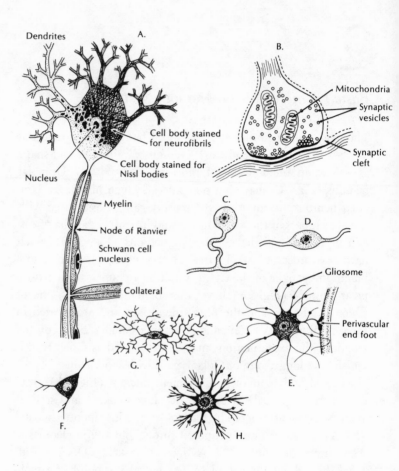

3. Histology of Nervous Tissue
A. multipolar neuron   B. synapse   C. unipolar neuron   D. bipolar neuron   E. fibrous astrocyte   F. oligodendrocyte   G. microglia   H. protoplasmic astrocyte

They are readily demonstrated with basic aniline dyes. They are known to be composed of nucleoproteins and iron. Electron micrographs reveal Nissl bodies to be made up of a series of parallel membranes (cisternae) which may anastomose. The membranes contain RNA granules (ribosomal RNA and protein). Nissl bodies appear to be condensations of granular endoplasmic reticulum which is commonly found in protein-producing cells. The function of the Nissl bodies is not fully understood, but they probably play an important role in protein synthesis. When the neuron is injured the Nissl substance undergoes dissolution, a process known as chromatolysis. If recovery ensues the Nissl substance first reappears around the nuclear membrane. It is probably formed from material in the nucleus. Nissl substance is depleted during the chronic stimulation of the cell.

Other intracellular structures found in all neurons are neurofibrils, which extend throughout the cytoplasm, dendrites, and axon. They are best demonstrated by metallic impregnation techniques, e.g. silver. There is no exact counterpart of neurofibrils in electron micrographs. They probably are condensations of small tubular elements known as microtubules and neurofilaments. The function of neurofibrils is not fully understood, but they may be concerned with metabolism, the transport of materials, and structural support.

Mitochondria are found throughout the cytoplasm, dendrites, and axon and are particularly concentrated at the terminal ends of nerve fibers. Their structure and function are similar to those found in other cell types. They are spherical or elongated and are composed of unit membranes formed of phospholipids combined with protein. Mitochondria are double membranous structures with the inner layer thrown into folds called cristae. Associated with the outer aspects of the inner membrane are the enzymes for the tricarboxylic acid cycle. On the inner aspect are the enzymes for the cytochrome electron transfer system. They are, therefore, the site for aerobic respiration in the cell. Current

9

research indicates that within the matrix of mitochondria there may be other enzyme systems.

A Golgi apparatus is found within the nerve cell cytoplasm. This is a fine reticular network of unit membranes in the form of flattened sacs, and large and small vesicles. In other cells the Golgi apparatus is concerned with the storage and packaging of secretion droplets. It may have a similar function in nerve cells. It is very sensitive to nerve cell injury, undergoing fragmentation and dissolution before the Nissl substance.

Other cytoplasmic inclusions and organelles found in nerve cells are vacuoles, fatty substances, melanin pigment (confined to specific cells), lysosomes, and lipochrome pigment. The last increases with age.

A neuron may have one dendrite or many. The dendrite is usually short but branches profusely and at any angle. It is attached to the cell body by a broad base but tapers in diameter rapidly. Dendrites contain Nissl substance and mitochondria. They conduct toward the cell body. Dendrites are in synaptic relation with the terminal ends of a large number of axons.

In contrast to the dendrite the axon is usually long and does not taper. There is only one to a cell. The axon is devoid of Nissl substance but does contain mitochondria and many neurofibrils. Branches of the axon are few in number except at the terminal end. Those that come off in the course of the fiber are called collaterals. They arise at right angles at the nodes of Ranvier. The axon conducts the impulse away from the cell body.

The axon may have one or two coverings: myelin and sheath of Schwann (Fig. 4). The actual extension of the cell body is known as the axis cylinder, and surrounding this may be a lipoid material, myelin, which appears in concentric lamellae. In the peripheral nervous system, and also centrally, the myelin is broken into segments by the nodes of Ranvier, which are the points where the axis cylinder is devoid of myelin. Outside the myelin sheath in the peripheral nervous system is found a single

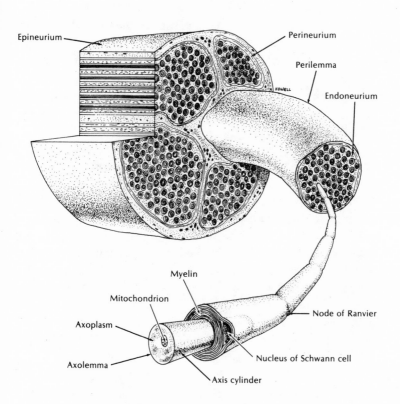

Epineurium
Perineurium
Perilemma
Endoneurium
HOWELL
Myelin
Mitochondrion
Axoplasm
Node of Ranvier
Axolemma
Nucleus of Schwann cell
Axis cylinder

4. Cross Section of a Peripheral Nerve

11

cell layered membrane, the sheath of Schwann. The Schwann cell contains a scanty amount of cytoplasm but a prominent nucleus. One sheath cell occupies one internodal space. In light microscopy a thin tubular sheath, the neurilemma, surrounds the nerve fiber. Electron micrographs reveal this to be the cell membrane of the Schwann cell. It is believed that the Schwann cell forms the myelin as it circumnavigates the axis cylinder by laying down concentric lamellae, formed largely from plasma membranes of the Schwann cell. In the central nervous system this function is subserved by specialized cells called oligodendrocytes. At the terminal end of the axon the sheaths are lost and the fiber branches at all angles forming terminal naked fibers called telodendria.

The synapse (Fig. 3B) is the junction between the terminal ends of an axon of one neuron and the dendrites or cell body of another. Synaptic endings have also been described in relation to the naked proximal and distal ends of the axon, and between dendrites. Protoplasmic continuity does not exist at the synapse but there is contiguity. Electron microscopists have described a synaptic cleft between the thickened presynaptic and subsynaptic membranes of about 200 Å.

Synaptic terminals may take on various forms. A common form is a ball-like ending known as a bouton. Other types are basket endings, knobs, spines, and rings. The presynaptic endings contain mitochondria and synaptic vesicles. The latter contains the chemical mediator which may be released into the synaptic cleft upon arrival of an impulse. The synapse is polarized; conduction is from the axon of one neuron to the dendrites or cell body of another.

The cell body is the site of the synthesis of certain substances such as transmitter molecules, macromolecules, vesicle membranes, and various enzymes. These are transported throughout the cell and processes. This may be over great distances in the axon. Axonal transport may be slow (1 mm/day) or fast (100–

400 mm/day). In this manner the transmitter substance reaches the synaptic ending where it is stored in vesicles until its release into the synaptic cleft. Retrograde transport of materials such as small enzymes picked up by the axon terminal also occurs.

Over thirty different substances have been implicated as transmitters, many of which are putative in that they do not meet all the criteria required to classify as transmitters at the present time. Transmitters fall into four general categories: acetylcholine, catecholamines, amino acids, and peptides. Acetylcholine has been recognized as a transmitter for a long time, and consequently has been the subject of considerable investigation. The catecholamines include norepinephrine, dopamine, serotonin, and histamine. Among the amino acids are GABA (gamma-aminobutyric acid), glutamic acid, glycine, and taurine. A large number of peptides may be putative transmitters such as the enkephalins and endorphins, substance P, neurotensin, and angiotensin.

After the release of the transmitter into the synaptic cleft it diffuses across the cleft to bind with a molecular receptor. This results in depolarization or hyperpolarization of the postsynaptic membrane. The transmitter is then cleared from the cleft by enzymatic deactivation, reuptake by the presynaptic ending, uptake by glial cells, or diffusion.

In some areas of the brain such as the vestibular nuclei, electrical synapses have been described. These are gap junctions where the two membranes are closely opposed. There is usually a space of no more than 40 Å. This constitutes a low-resistance electrical pathway between two neurons.

When an axon is cut (axotomy) changes occur in both the cell body and axon, particularly distal to the transection. The cell body swells and the Nissl bodies undergo dissolution—a process known as chromatolysis. The nucleus is usually displaced to the periphery. These changes are reversible if regeneration occurs. The axis cylinder and myelin distal to the cut undergo swelling

13

and fragmentation, producing degenerated products which are removed by macrophages. The Schwann cells increase in number and form bands within the endoneurial tube and bridge the area of the cut.

In the peripheral nervous system regeneration may occur. The tip of the severed axon sprouts a number of fine branches which attempt to find a Schwann cell band and follow it through the distal endoneurial tube. A number may succeed in doing so. Those that fail degenerate. Upon reaching an appropriate end organ they effect a functional connection. Those that do not attain the proper receptor or effector also degenerate. During the growth of the axon the Schwann cells reconstitute the myelin so that the nerve fiber approaches its former diameter.

In the central nervous system regeneration does not occur, although sprouting of the severed axon tip takes place. However, growth of the sprouts is subsequently aborted. This may be due to a rapid deposition of glia that form a scar which blocks the regenerating fiber. Another factor may be the absence of Schwann cells, which in the peripheral nervous system form bands that serve as guides for the regenerating fiber.

Although regeneration does not occur in the central nervous system collateral sprouting does take place. Following transection of a central nerve fiber, intact parallel fibers may exhibit sprouting at the nodes of Ranvier. These branches find their way into the pathway of the degenerating fiber and eventually effect a functional connection. The phenomenon of collateral sprouting also occurs in the peripheral nervous system.

Other elements found within the central nervous system are the neuroglia, comprised of astrocytes, oligodendrocytes, and microglia. Astrocytes, arising from ectoderm, are divided into two types, fibrous and protoplasmic. Both types are found in gray and white matter though the fibrous type is more numerous in the white matter and the protoplasmic type in the gray. The fibrous astrocytes (Fig. 3E) contain numerous fibrous processes which rarely branch. The cell body contains an oval nucleus with little chromatin. There is also very little cytoplasm. The processes contain granules called gliosomes. These are apparently the sites of mitochondria. Some of the processes have expansions around blood vessels known as perivascular end feet. The fibers also form a network around the nerve cells. Fibrous astrocytes are found in large numbers at the surface of the central nervous system, where, with the pia mater, they form the pial-glial membrane. Protoplasmic astrocytes (Fig. 3H) contain numerous thick processes which branch profusely. The processes have gliosomes and perivascular end feet. The nucleus has the same appearance as the fibrous astrocytes, but the cell body contains more cytoplasm. All astrocytes are characterized by numerous small fibrils extending through the cytoplasm. The fibrous type, however, contains more of these elements.

Oligodendrocytes (Fig. 3F), which are also derived from ectoderm, are smaller than astrocytes and are found in both gray and white matter. In the gray matter they frequently are found as satellites to neurons. In the white matter they are located along the course of the nerve fibers. Oligodendrocytes have a few slender processes with few branches. There are no perivascular end feet, but gliosomes are present. The nucleus stains darker than in astrocytes and the cytoplasm is scanty.

Microglia (Fig. 3G) are of mesodermal origin. They are probably part of the reticulo-endothelial system since they revert to phagocytes following injury to the nervous system. The cells are very small and have delicate tortuous processes. They are found in both gray and white matter, and the cell body varies considerably in shape.

The ependyma is composed of a single layer of cuboidal cells lining the central canal of the spinal cord and ventricles of the brain. At certain locations within each of the ventricles blood vessels and connective tissue of the pia mater push the ependyma ahead into the ventricles forming the choroid plexuses. The choroid plexuses play a role in the production and absorption of cerebrospinal fluid which will be discussed in Chapter 20.

The neuroglia have a number of functions and have long been recognized as supportive. The receptive areas (synaptic zone) of neurons are ensheathed by astrocytic processes. This has led to speculation that astrocytes may serve as insulators of synaptic surfaces. Following injury to the nervous system the glia proliferate to fill in and wall off the defect forming a glial scar. If the area is large a cyst may form with a glial membrane as the wall. The role played by the astrocytes in the blood brain barrier is a controversial one. This will be discussed in Chapter 21. Recently contacts have been described between glia and nerve cells and glia and glia, and it has been speculated that glia may be conductive since the contacts might be a mechanism for electrotonic spread of potentials. Finally, as stated above, oligodendrocytes play an important role in the formation of myelin in the central nervous system.

Peripheral nerves contain a variable number of nerve fibers. Usually within each nerve the fibers are organized into several bundles known as fascicles (Fig. 4). Each fascicle is surrounded by a selectively permeable cellular membrane called the perilemma or perineural epithelium. Within each fascicle are myelinated and nonmyelinated fibers supported by a delicate connective tissue known as the endoneurium. Immediately outside the perilemma is the perineurium, which is a dense connective tissue composed of elastic and collagenous fibers and containing numerous blood vessels and lymphatics. All the fascicles are bound together into one nerve trunk by the epineurium, which is a loose connective tissue containing collagenous and elastic fibers, fat, and blood vessels. It blends in with the connective tissue of the surrounding structures. The endoneurium, perineurium, and epineurium are derived from the mesoderm.

A single nerve fiber may be afferent or efferent and be concerned with either the soma or viscera. This results in four functional components of peripheral nerves. General somatic afferent (GSA) fibers convey afferent impulses from the general soma such as the skin, bone, skeletal muscle, joints, ligaments, tendons, etc. General visceral afferent (GVA) fibers arise from receptors in the viscera, including blood vessels. General somatic efferent (GSE) fibers innervate skeletal muscles derived from myotomes. General visceral efferent (GVE) fibers belong to the autonomic nervous system and supply smooth and cardiac muscles and glands.

Generally, all spinal nerves contain these components. In the cranial nerves there may be three additional components due to the presence of special sense organs and skeletal muscle derived from branchial arches. Nerve fibers supplying the branchial muscles are referred to as special visceral efferent (SVE). Special visceral afferent (SVA) fibers arise from the chemical receptors of taste and smell, whereas the special somatic afferent (SSA) component is associated with the special sense of sight and receptors in the inner ear.

No cranial nerve has all seven components. The components of each of the cranial nerves are listed in the chart on pp. 18-19. In addition, the oculomotor, trochlear, abducens, and hypoglossal may contain proprioceptive fibers which are GSA.

Within the central nervous system each functional component is usually represented by a column of cells which may or may not be discontinuous throughout the neuraxis. Thus, as a peripheral nerve approaches the central nervous system its individual functional components separate out and terminate in (afferent) or arise from (efferent) a nucleus belonging to the column related to its function.

17

I	Olfactory	SVA	From receptors in the olfactory membrane in the roof of the nasal cavity
II	Optic	SSA	From ganglion cells in the retina
III	Oculomotor	GSE	To inferior, medial, and superior recti; inferior oblique, and levator palpebrae superioris (myotome origin)
		GVE	Preganglionic parasympathetic to ciliary ganglion. Postganglionic to ciliary muscle and sphincter of pupil
IV	Trochlear	GSE	To superior oblique muscle (myotome origin)
V	Trigeminal	GSA	Main general sensory nerve of the head, e.g. skin, paranasal sinuses, oral and nasal cavities, etc.
		SVE	To muscles of mastication and the anterior belly of the digastric, mylohyoid, tensor tympani, and tensor veli palatini (branchial arch origin)
VI	Abducens	GSE	To lateral rectus muscle (myotome origin)
VII	Facial	SVE	To facial muscles, including buccinator, posterior belly of the digastric, stapedius, and stylohyoid (branchial arch origin)
		SVA	From taste buds on anterior two-thirds of tongue
		GVE	Preganglionic parasympathetic to sphenopalatine and submandibular ganglia. Postganglionics to lacrimal, submandibular, and sublingual glands

		GVA	From mucous membrane in area of the palate
		GSA	From skin of external ear
VIII	Auditory	SSA	From hair cells in the inner ear (cochlear and vestibular)
IX	Glossopharyngeal	SVE	To stylopharyngeus muscle (branchial arch origin)
		SVA	From taste buds on posterior third of tongue
		GVE	Preganglionic parasympathetic to otic ganglion. Postganglionics to parotid gland
		GVA	From mucous membrane of pharynx
		GSA	From skin of external ear
X	Vagus	SVE	To muscles of the pharynx, larynx, and esophagus (branchial arch origin)
		SVA	From taste buds on epiglottis
		GVE	Preganglionic parasympathetics to ganglia in thoracic and abdominal cavities. Postganglionics to adjacent visceral structures
		GVA	From mucous membrane of thoracic and abdominal viscera
		GSA	From skin of external ear and meninges of the posterior cranial fossa
XI	Spinal accessory	SVE	To sternocleidomastoid and trapezius muscles (branchial arch origin)
XII	Hypoglossal	GSE	To muscles of tongue (myotome origin)

19

3

Basic Neural Mechanisms

In the spinal cord the gray matter which contains cell bodies is arranged in a central H-shaped mass (Fig. 5C). Peripheral to this is the white matter, made up largely of myelinated fibers. The gray matter is composed of aggregates of cell bodies known as nuclei. The neurons making up a nucleus generally have similar connections and functions. Entering the spinal cord at the apex of the dorsal horn of the gray matter is the dorsal root of the spinal nerve. The cell bodies of these fibers are unipolar and are located in the dorsal root ganglion. A ganglion is an aggregate of cell bodies outside the central nervous system. The ventral root exits from the base of the ventral horn of the gray matter. The cell bodies of these fibers are multipolar and located in the ventral horn.

The white matter is divided into three masses of fibers known as funiculi. The dorsal funiculus is located between the dorsal midline and dorsal root, the lateral funiculus between the dorsal and ventral roots, and the ventral funiculus between the ventral root and ventral midline. Within each funiculus are found bundles of fibers called fasciculi or tracts. The fibers within a fasciculus usually have a common origin, termination, and function. They may be either ascending or descending.

The division of the gray matter of the spinal cord into Rexed's laminae makes for a convenient reference map in desig-

20

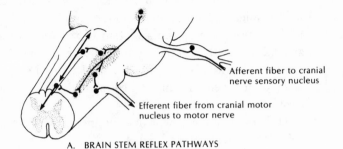

Afferent fiber to cranial
nerve sensory nucleus

Efferent fiber from cranial motor
nucleus to motor nerve

A. BRAIN STEM REFLEX PATHWAYS

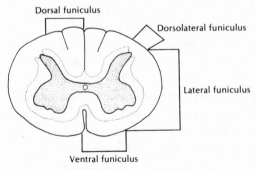

Dorsal root

Dorsal root ganglion

Afferent fiber

Efferent fiber

Spinal nerve

Ventral root

B. SPINAL CORD REFLEX PATHWAYS

Dorsal funiculus

Dorsolateral funiculus

Lateral funiculus

Ventral funiculus

C. SPINAL CORD CROSS SECTION

5. Reflex Pathways

21

nating precise points within the gray (Fig. 6). This is based on cytological differences and may reflect functional differences as well. Laminae I through VI are in the dorsal horn, VII includes the intermediate gray and a portion of the ventral horn, VIII and IX are in the ventral horn, and X is around the central canal and consists largely of neuroglia. Lamina IX contains the large motor neurons and II corresponds to the substantia gelatinosa.

The orderly arrangement of gray and white matter remains constant throughout the spinal cord, varying only in relative mass. The volume of gray matter reflects the size of the spinal nerve associated with that level. Thus its size is markedly increased at the cervical and lumbosacral segments of the spinal cord for the innervation of upper and lower extremities respectively. The white matter increases in absolute mass from caudal to rostral levels of the spinal cord due to the progressive accumulation of fibers in ascending fasciculi and a gradual diminution of fibers in descending tracts. In the brain, due to factors which will be discussed later, the gray matter and white matter intermingle. More or less discrete nuclei and fasciculi appear usually at the periphery of the brain stem. The central core contains diffuse tracts and nuclei and is known as the reticular formation. The cranial nerves do not show the constant pattern of dorsal and ventral roots as is the case of the spinal nerves—they may be either purely sensory or motor. If the nerve is mixed the fibers usually enter and leave the brain stem in the same root. Centrally, the nuclei associated with cranial nerves are arranged in functional columns; the fibers separate centrally and arise or terminate in the appropriate column.

The reflex arc usually consists of a receptor, afferent neuron, intercalated neuron (association or internuncial), efferent neuron, and effector. In a few instances (the stretch or myotatic reflex) the intercalated neuron may be absent. The recep-

22

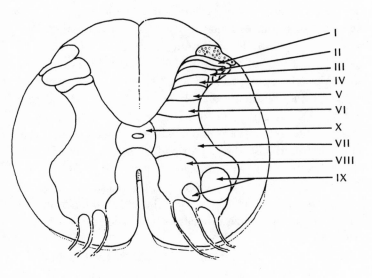

I
II
III
IV
V
VI
X
VII
VIII
IX

6. Laminae of Rexed

tors vary considerably in complexity from naked nerve endings to complicated receptor organs like the retina and organ of Corti. The receptor responding to an adequate stimulus sets up an impulse in the afferent neuron whose cell body is located in the dorsal root ganglion or one of the ganglia of the cranial nerves. The afferent neuron conveys the impulse centrally via the dorsal root of the spinal nerve or one of the cranial nerves. Upon entering the spinal cord (Fig. 5B) the fibers of the dorsal root bifurcate into ascending and descending limbs. Some of the fibers ascend in the dorsal funiculus to the medulla where they synapse in nuclei found at that level. These will be discussed in Chapter 5. The remaining fibers course up and down a variable number of segments and terminate in synaptic relationships with neurons found in all laminae of the gray matter. Those that terminate directly on the large motor neurons in lamina IX take part in the formation of the myotatic or stretch reflex. These reflexes are monosynaptic. Neurons in other laminae may synapse directly or indirectly (by way of other intercalated neurons) with efferent neurons of the ventral horn. The efferent neuron whose cell body is located in lamina IX of the ventral horn will exit by way of the ventral root or one of the cranial nerves, ending in relation to an effector, which may be either a muscle or gland.

The course and termination of the intercalated neuron determines the pattern of the reflex response. The intercalated neuron may ascend or descend a number of segments, resulting in an intersegmental reflex. If the intercalated neuron is confined to the same segment into which the afferent fiber enters, the result will be an intrasegmental reflex. The intercalated neuron may cross to the opposite side, resulting in a crossed or contralateral reflex. In this case the intercalated neuron is referred to as commissural. Many of the axons of intercalated neurons ascend and descend for a considerable distance in a band of fibers surrounding the gray matter. This

24

group of fibers is referred to as the fasciculus proprius or fasciculus spinospinalis. Other spinal reflex tracts are the septomarginal fasciculus, located in the dorsal funiculus adjacent to the median sulcus, and the fasciculus interfascicularis, or comma bundle, located in relationship to the intermediate septum of the dorsal funiculus. These tracts contain ascending and descending limbs of the dorsal root fibers. They ultimately terminate on internuncial neurons.

Afferent fibers of cranial nerves terminate in specific nuclei (Fig. 5A). Neurons within these nuclei may constitute intercalated neurons of reflex arcs. These fibers may pass directly to motor nuclei, ascend or descend in specific fasciculi, or enter the reticular formation. The last is continuous with the fasciculus proprius of the spinal cord. Over this pathway may be mediated many of the reflexes involving spinal and cranial nerves.

Before proceeding to a detailed discussion of specific sensory pathways it may be profitable to first point out those features common to all such systems (Fig. 7). The exceptions to the general pattern presented will be pointed out as the specific pathways are discussed. The cell body of the primary (sensory) neuron is located in a ganglion which is outside the central nervous system. The peripheral process of the neuron is incorporated in a spinal or cranial nerve and terminates in relation to a receptor. The receptors respond to various stimuli and set up an impulse in the afferent fiber. The central process of the neuron enters the spinal cord or brain stem and bifurcates into ascending and descending limbs, which extend for variable distances. Throughout their course numerous collaterals are given off. Sensory fibers terminate in relation to a secondary neuron found in a nucleus located in the central nervous system. The secondary neuron may project cephalically as a continuation of a conscious pathway or to higher integrative centers. It may also, as an internuncial neuron,

25

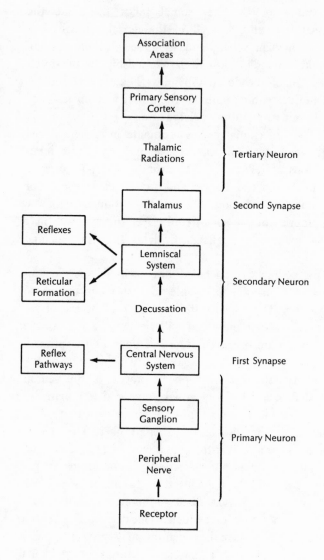

7. General Principles of Sensory Pathways

26

terminate either directly or by way of other internuncial neurons on a motor neuron. The motor neuron leaves the central nervous system via a peripheral nerve to end in an effector, forming the basis for a simple reflex arc.

If the secondary neuron is involved in the conscious pathway, it crosses the midline at the level of its origin and forms a lemniscus on the opposite side, and continues uninterrupted to terminate on a tertiary neuron in the thalamus, a division of the diencephalon. In its course the secondary neuron sends collaterals and terminals into the reticular formation and tectum. The tertiary neuron sends its axon via the internal capsule and corona radiata as thalamic radiations to terminate in the appropriate primary sensory cortex. The primary cortex is connected with cortical association areas, where the sensation is interpreted, integrated, and modified.

4

Pain, Temperature, and Tactile Pathways

The general features of sensory systems have been covered, and now the pain, temperature, and tactile pathways will be described. The receptors for these pathways are naked nerve endings and simple encapsulated organs (Fig. 8). A poorly myelinated or nonmyelinated fiber branches profusely and ends as a naked terminal among the epithelial cells of the skin and viscera, in subcutaneous tissue, and in the walls of blood vessels. These naked nerve endings are the nociceptors, but many are also polymodal in that they may respond to thermal and mechanical stimulation. Some fibers terminate in a cup-like expansion in relation to a specialized epithelial cell. These are thought to be mechanoreceptors (Merkel's tactile disc), which respond to light touch. Other tactile receptors are the peritrichial endings, which are naked fibers forming a basket-like arrangement around the hair follicles. The ability to detect temperature change is probably also a function of the naked nerve endings.

The fibers of the peripheral nerves, which convey impulses originating in the receptors cited above, are poorly myelinated (A delta fibers) or nonmyelinated (C fibers). Their cell bodies are small, unipolar, and located in the cerebrospinal ganglia. In the spinal nerves the central processes of these cells separate from other fibers of the dorsal root to make up its lateral division, and upon entering the spinal cord they bifurcate and

28

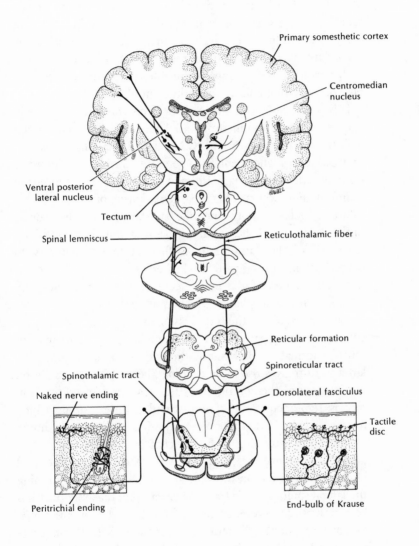

Primary somesthetic cortex

Centromedian nucleus

Ventral posterior lateral nucleus

Tectum

Spinal lemniscus

Reticulothalamic fiber

Reticular formation

Spinothalamic tract

Spinoreticular tract

Naked nerve ending

Dorsolateral fasciculus

Tactile disc

Peritrichial ending

End-bulb of Krause

8. Pain, Temperature, and Tactile Pathways

29

ascend or descend in the dorsolateral fasciculus (zone of Lissauer) for only a few segments. The fibers and the numerous collaterals terminate in the gray matter of the dorsal horn. Secondary fibers arising from these nuclei make connections with various nuclear groups within the spinal cord for the purpose of mediating reflexes, as outlined in Chapter 3.

It is probable that C and A delta fibers concerned with pain and temperature terminate in all laminae of the gray matter with the exception of IX and X. Not all these laminae, however, project on to higher centers. There are considerable interconnections within the gray matter where a great deal of processing of information occurs. This is particularly true of lamina II, the substantia gelatinosa. The peptide, substance P, which is found in the small cells of the dorsal root ganglia and also particularly lamina II of the dorsal horn, is thought to be excitatory to neurons transmitting pain to higher centers. On the other hand, stimulation of the periaqueductal gray of the midbrain, an area rich in enkephalin, which is an endogenous morphine-like substance, blocks the transmission of pain. This probably involves descending pathways from the midbrain to the brain stem reticular formation, particularly the nucleus raphe magnus. The latter in turn gives rise to descending fibers which terminate on interneurons of the dorsal horn. Although this descending pathway is serotonergic, the fibers stimulate interneurons which release enkephalin that blocks transmission in the pain pathway.

Pain fibers ascending to higher centers seem to arise principally from laminae I, V, VII, and VIII. Most cross at the level of origin and ascend in the ventral and lateral funiculi forming the lateral spinothalamic tract. A ventral spinothalamic tract has been described; however since the fibers have the same termination and function, designating two separate tracts is not necessary. The term "spinal lemniscus" is frequently used to indicate the spinothalamic tract. The tract terminates in the thalamus but has other endings particularly in the reticular formation and tectum.

Lamination occurs in the tract in the sense that the first fibers entering the tract and representing sacral levels are the most lateral and dorsal. Fibers entering at successively higher levels assume a more medial and ventral position. Throughout the medulla and pons the tract maintains a lateral position. It then migrates dorsally in the midbrain and, upon reaching diencephalic levels, turns laterally to terminate in the ventral posterior lateral nucleus, the posterior nuclei, and the nonspecific thalamic nuclei (intralaminar, parafascicular, and centromedian). The ventral posterior lateral nucleus projects fibers as general thalamic radiations through the internal capsule and corona radiata to terminate in the postcentral gyrus, which constitutes the primary sensory cortex. The primary cortex has extensive connections with association areas where the sensation is interpreted and integrated with other incoming information.

The spinoreticular component of the spinothalamic tract terminates in pools of neurons in the brain stem reticular formation, particularly the medial portion. The reticular formation gives rise to a reticulothalamic system which terminates in the nonspecific thalamic and posterior nuclei. Thus there is also a spinoreticulothalamic pathway for pain. This is multisynaptic and partially uncrossed. It is also a slow conducting pathway. The spinothalamic fibers terminating in the ventral posterior lateral nucleus are referred to as the neospinothalamic tract and are concerned with the appreciation of sharp, pricking, well localized, and short-duration pain and probably temperature. These are mediated by the A delta fibers. A projection to the cerebral cortex is also necessary for further elaboration. The fibers terminating directly in the nonspecific nuclei are referred to as the paleospinothalamic tract. These, along with the spinoreticulothalamic system, archispinothalamic tract, are con-

31

cerned with dull, aching, poorly localized and persistent pain. These modalities are conveyed by the C fibers in the peripheral nervous system. Since the thalamus is the lowest level of sensory appreciation, it is this type of pain which may be realized at the thalamic level.

A number of clinical conditions demonstrate the anatomy of the pain and temperature pathway. In cases of intractable pain the lateral spinothalamic tract may be sectioned in the spinal cord, the operation of cordotomy. However, the sensation of pain may return in one or two years as a result of the diffuse nature of the tract's pathways. The inability to perceive pain and detect temperature change is on the opposite side of the body, and will extend as high as a few segments below the level of the section. This is due to the fact that when the dorsal root fibers enter they ascend and descend for a few segments. If the tract is involved in a lesion in the brain stem there is a complete loss of sense of pain and temperature change on the opposite side of the body. A degenerative condition known as syringomyelia begins around the central canal, usually in the cervical enlargement, with interruption of the ventral white commissure which conveys pain and temperature fibers from the dorsal horn across the midline. The first sign is a bilateral segmental loss of sense of pain and temperature change in the upper extremities.

5

Proprioception, Tactile Discrimination, and Stereognosis

This system includes the sense of position and movement (proprioception), two-point discrimination, vibratory sense, and stereognosis (three-dimensional sense). The receptors for this system are much more complicated than those for pain and temperature. The system contains several types of encapsulated organs (Meissner's, Golgi-Mazzoni, and Pacinian corpuscles) which vary in size, shape, and manner of fiber termination (Fig. 9). In each case a myelinated fiber loses its myelin upon entering the core of the receptor. The connective tissue of the peripheral nerve blends with the connective tissue capsule.

Meissner's corpuscle is elongated and contains a thin connective-tissue capsule. The nerve fiber, upon entering the gelatinous core, spirals and branches considerably. The fibers terminate as swellings in relation to flattened cells. The Golgi-Mazzoni corpuscle is small and spherical. The capsule is slightly thicker than Meissner's, the nerve fiber is less coiled, and branching is sparse. The Pacinian corpuscle is the largest of the group, measuring from 1–4 mm in length. It is oval in shape with a very heavy capsule. The fiber continues to the distal end of the core, ends in a knob, and may give off a few short branches en route. Nerve fibers have been observed to pass through a corpuscle to enter another. The Pacinian cor-

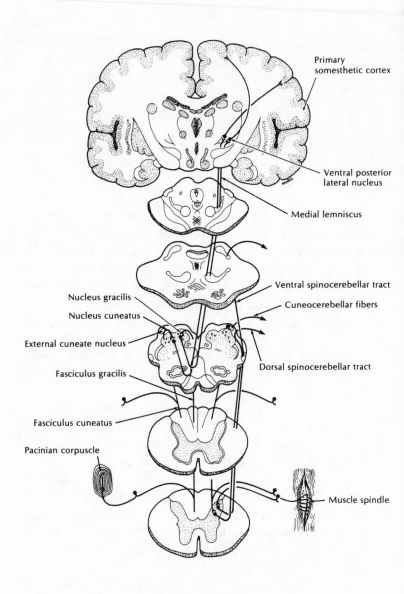

Primary
somesthetic cortex

Ventral posterior
lateral nucleus

Medial lemniscus

Ventral spinocerebellar tract

Cuneocerebellar fibers

Nucleus gracilis

Nucleus cuneatus

External cuneate nucleus

Dorsal spinocerebellar tract

Fasciculus gracilis

Fasciculus cuneatus

Pacinian corpuscle

Muscle spindle

9. Proprioception and Two-Point Discrimination Pathways

puscles, which are located in the dermis, in the superficial fascia, in the proximity of blood vessels, and in the viscera, are touch, pressure, and vibratory receptors.

Within muscle and tendon there are complex receptors known as muscle spindles and Golgi tendon organs. These monitor tension, length of the muscle, and rate of contraction. The muscle spindle (Fig. 10) is found in parallel with the extrafusal fibers of skeletal muscle. It is fusiform in shape and contains a variable number of modified muscle fibers, the intrafusal fibers. These are surrounded by a thin capsule. The intrafusal fibers are of two types: nuclear bag and nuclear chain. The noncontractile equatorial region of the nuclear bag fiber is enlarged and contains a large number of nuclei. The nuclear chain fiber is slender and of uniform diameter. The nuclei are arranged end-to-end.

Two types of sensory fibers enter the spindle. Group IA fibers terminate in a spiral arrangement around the equator of the nuclear bag fiber and to a lesser extent around the nuclear chain fiber. These are the primary sensory or annulospiral endings. Group II fibers terminate at the polar regions by spraying out on the surface of the fiber. These are the secondary or flower spray endings. A thinly myelinated motor fiber also enters the spindle. This terminates on the polar regions of the intrafusal fibers and is known as the gamma efferent. The extrafusal fibers of the muscle are innervated by large alpha motor neurons. The Golgi tendon organs are supplied by group IB fibers. These terminate as leaf-like expansions between bundles of collagenous fibers of tendons usually at or near the junction of muscle and tendon.

When a muscle is passively stretched the sensory endings on the intrafusal fibers are stimulated. The sensory fibers synapse directly with large motor neurons of lamina IX. The result is a contraction of the muscle, the stretch reflex. The spindle is shortened and the receptors cease to discharge. If the tension is

35

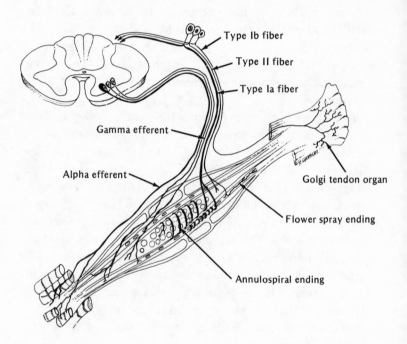

Type Ib fiber

Type II fiber

Type Ia fiber

Gamma efferent

Alpha efferent

Golgi tendon organ

Flower spray ending

Annulospiral ending

10. Muscle Spindle

36

to be maintained the gamma efferent must fire to bring about contraction of the intrafusal fibers, thus continuing the stimulation of the sensory endings. The gamma efferent is under both reflex control and control from higher centers. When a muscle contracts or is stretched the Golgi tendon organs discharge. These receptors are thought to measure tension.

All spinal nerves and many of the cranial nerves carry fibers which convey proprioceptive and tactile impulses. The fibers are relatively large and well myelinated and conduct at a rapid rate. The cell bodies, located in the dorsal root ganglia or the ganglia of cranial nerves, are large as compared with those for pain. The fibers of the spinal nerves conveying the impulses enter the spinal cord by way of the medial division of the dorsal root. They enter the dorsal funiculus where they bifurcate into ascending and descending limbs. Some of these fibers may enter one of the reflex pathways located in the dorsal funiculus (fasciculus interfascicularis or septomarginal fasciculus) and eventually effect a reflex connection with neurons in the dorsal and intermediate gray or, in the case of the myotatic reflex, directly on the ventral horn cell.

A lamination occurs in the dorsal funiculus in that the fibers entering at the lowest level (sacral fibers) assume a position adjacent to the dorsomedial septum. As more and more fibers enter, they take up a more lateral position. The cervical fibers are therefore the most lateral of the group. Upon attaining the midthoracic region a septum begins to appear in the dorsal funiculus. This, the dorsal intermediate septum, separates the dorsal funiculus into two fasciculi. The medial group of fibers is referred to as the fasciculus gracilis. It contains fibers which have entered via the sacral, lumbar, and lower thoracic nerves. The lateral group is called the fasciculus cuneatus. Fibers which make up this fasciculus enter at upper thoracic and cervical levels. The fibers of these two fasciculi terminate in corresponding nuclei in the medulla,

37

the nucleus gracilis and the nucleus cuneatus (dorsal column nuclei). This constitutes the first synapse in the pathway to the cerebral cortex.

Secondary fibers arising from these nuclei cross the midline in a sweeping arc and are referred to as internal arcuate fibers. Upon attaining the opposite side they ascend adjacent to the midline in a tract called the medial lemniscus. Throughout the medulla the medial lemniscus is situated adjacent to the midline, and upon reaching the pons it migrates laterally, assuming the shape of a horizontal band. In the upper portion of the pons it begins to pass dorsolaterally and continues in this position into the midbrain. When the thalamus is reached it passes into the ventral posterior lateral nucleus, where the fibers terminate. This constitutes the second synapse in this pathway. Tertiary fibers arise from this nucleus and ascend via the internal capsule and corona radiata to terminate in the cortex of the postcentral gyrus. This area constitutes the primary somesthetic cortex. It has extensive connections with adjacent association cortex.

Some of the primary fibers coursing in the dorsal funiculus terminate in the nucleus dorsalis (Clarke's column) located in lamina VII of the thoracic and upper lumbar cord. These cells receive terminals from fibers entering via the sacral, lumbar, and lower thoracic dorsal roots. The axons of the cells in this nucleus ascend as the dorsal spinocerebellar tract in the dorsolateral portion of the lateral funiculus of the same side. They continue into the medulla, where they enter the restiform body (inferior cerebellar peduncle), and then pass by way of this peduncle to terminate principally in the vermis portion of the cerebellar cortex. Other cells in lamina VII of the lumbar cord give rise to the ventral spinocerebellar tract. The fibers which terminate among these cells are for the most part interneurons conveying information from the lower half of the body. The ventral spinocerebellar tract is largely crossed. This tract ascends peripheral to the lateral spinothalamic tract through the cord, medulla, and pons. Upon reaching the upper levels of the pons, it enters the brachium conjunctivum (superior cerebellar peduncle), and then enters the cerebellum to terminate in the cortex of the vermis. Lateral to the nucleus cuneatus in the medulla is located a mass of neurons whose cytology is similar to those of the nucleus dorsalis in the cord. This nucleus is referred to as the external (lateral or accessory) cuneate nucleus. Many of the primary fibers of the fasciculus cuneatus terminate in this nucleus. Axons of secondary neurons arising from this nucleus enter the adjacent restiform body and also terminate in the vermis of the cerebellum. These are referred to as direct (dorsal) arcuate fibers. These three tracts, dorsal spinocerebellar tract, ventral spinocerebellar tract, and direct arcuate fibers, constitute important pathways for proprioception and tactile information from the skeletal muscles of the trunk to the cerebellum. The functional significance of this will be discussed in a later section.

Tabes dorsalis and pernicious anemia attack the dorsal funiculus, destroying the component fibers. Any interruption of the proprioceptive pathway will be manifested by a lack of knowledge of the position of the limbs, spatial discrimination, loss of vibratory sense, etc. The patient has to watch his feet to walk, since he is not aware of their position by way of proprioception. He also loses the sense of two-point discrimination and some vibratory sensibility. Lesions which interrupt the medial lemniscus may result in the same set of symptoms. Since the medial lemniscus is adjacent to many other important pathways, however, other symptoms referable to those pathways will also be present. It is to be remembered that a unilateral lesion of the dorsal funiculus will give rise to homolateral symptoms, whereas a unilateral lesion of the medial lemniscus will result in contralateral deficits.

6

Trigeminal Pathways

The trigeminal nerve is the principal somesthetic nerve of the head. It supplies all of the skin anterior to a line drawn from the crown through the ear to a point under the mandible. In addition, it supplies the meninges in the anterior and middle cranial fossae and the mucous membrane of the oral and nasal cavities, including the teeth and paranasal sinuses. The receptors associated with it are the same as those discussed in the preceding chapters. The cell bodies of these afferent fibers are identical to those found in the dorsal root ganglia. They are located in the trigeminal (semilunar or Gasserian) ganglion (Fig. 11). The peripheral processes of these ganglion cells are distributed via the three divisions of the nerve (ophthalmic, maxillary, and mandibular). The central processes gather in a single bundle called the sensory root of the trigeminal nerve. This root courses through the middle of the brachium pontis. Its fibers run at near right angles to those of the brachium. Upon reaching the medial portion of the brachium pontis, the sensory root bifurcates into ascending and descending divisions. Approximately half of the constituent fibers of the sensory root descend only. A few of the fibers only ascend. The remaining fibers of the sensory root bifurcate into ascending and descending limbs. The descending root is concerned primarily with pain, temperature, and light touch, while the ascending division serves proprioception, two-point discrimina-

40

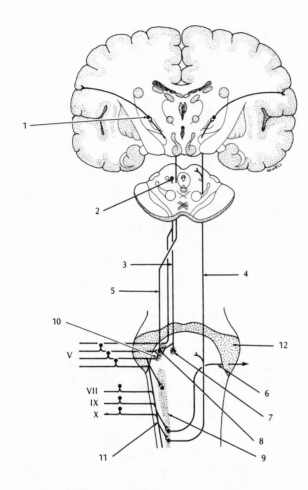

11. Trigeminal Connections

1. Ventral posterior medial nucleus   2. Mesencephalic nucleus of V
3. Mesencephalic tract of V   4. Ventral trigeminothalamic tract
5. Dorsal trigeminothalamic tract   6. Trigeminocerebellar fiber
7. Motor nucleus   8. Main sensory nucleus   9. Descending nucleus
10. Ascending root of V   11. Descending root of V   12. Inferior
cerebellar peduncle

41

tion, and light touch. The descending fibers continue through the lateral portion of the tegmentum of the pons, and into the lateral aspect of the medulla, and finally blend with the fibers of the zone of Lissauer in the upper cervical segments of the cord. Through the pons the descending root is covered laterally by the brachium pontis. In the upper half of the medulla it is covered by the restiform body. It reaches the surface in the lower medulla and upper cervical cord. Throughout the course of the descending root a nucleus, the descending nucleus of V, is located medial to the root. Fibers of the descending root terminate in all levels of the nucleus. Three subdivisions of the descending nucleus of V can be recognized. The subnucleus caudalis extends from the level of the caudal third of the inferior olive to C 3 or 4. The caudal nucleus and a portion of the reticular formation deep to it are homologous to laminae I through V of the dorsal horn. The subnucleus interpolaris is found at the level of the middle third of the inferior olive, and the subnucleus rostralis extends from this point to the level of entrance of the trigeminal nerve. These nuclei are probably homologous to the deeper laminae of the spinal cord gray matter. The small fibers of the trigeminal nerve descend only, terminate in the subnucleus caudalis, and are concerned with pain and temperature. Those fibers which bifurcate terminate at all levels of the descending nucleus as well as in the main sensory nucleus which is associated with the ascending root, and are thought to be for light touch or poorly localized tactile sensibility. The larger fibers which ascend only terminate in the main sensory nucleus and are related to discriminatory touch. This nucleus is similar to the dorsal column nuclei.

Secondary fibers arise from all levels of the descending nucleus, cross the midline, and ascend in a diffuse tract in the lateral portion of the medulla. This tract is called the trigeminal lemniscus (ventral trigeminothalamic tract). Throughout its course in the medulla and pons, numerous collaterals and terminals enter the reticular formation. In the upper pons the fibers intermingle with those of the medial lemniscus and accompany this tract into the thalamus. In the midbrain, fibers are given off to the tectum and tegmentum. The trigeminal lemniscus terminates in the ventral posterior medial nucleus and nonspecific nuclei of the thalamus. Tertiary fibers from the former nucleus project by way of the internal capsule and corona radiata to terminate in the postcentral gyrus. As in the case of the other systems, this gyrus has numerous connections with association areas.

The ascending root of the trigeminal nerve is short. Cells which intermingle with, and are located lateral to it, constitute the main sensory nucleus. The ascending root, whose fibers are for tactile discrimination, terminates in the main sensory nucleus. Secondary fibers from this nucleus ascend to the thalamus as the dorsal trigeminothalamic tract (dorsal division of the trigeminal lemniscus). Some fibers join the opposite trigeminal lemniscus. Others ascend on the same side ventral to the central gray of the midbrain. They terminate in the ventral posterior medial nucleus and subsequent connections with the cortex are the same as those described previously.

Proprioceptive fibers from the muscles of mastication also course with the trigeminal nerve. These fibers enter with the motor division, course adjacent to the motor and main sensory nuclei, and ascend in a bundle (mesencephalic root of V) to their cells of origin adjacent to the central gray of the midbrain. This is known as the mesencephalic nucleus of V. Its cells are unipolar, and their processes make up the mesencephalic tract. As the fibers pass the motor nucleus, collaterals, which are the same as the central processes of unipolar ganglion cells, are given off to this nucleus. This is the basis for a myotatic reflex involving the muscles of mastication. Other collaterals may enter the main sensory nucleus, and by this connection proprioception may reach higher conscious levels.

The main sensory and descending nuclei also send numerous fibers into the reticular formation bilaterally. This is in part a reflex path but also constitutes an important link in the trigeminoreticulothalamic pathway to the nonspecific thalamic nuclei. This is similar to the spinoreticulothalamic pathway for dull, diffuse pain from the trunk. The trigeminal nuclei, particularly the interpolaris and rostralis, also project to both sides of the cerebellum by way of the restiform body and probably by way of the brachium conjunctivum from the main sensory nucleus.

The facial, glossopharyngeal, and vagus nerves each has a general somatic afferent component. These fibers are distributed to the skin of the pinna and external auditory meatus of the external ear. In addition the vagus innervates the meninges in the posterior cranial fossa. The cell bodies of these fibers are unipolar and are located in the geniculate ganglion of VII, the superior ganglion of IX, and the jugular ganglion of X. The central processes of these cells enter the descending root of the trigeminal nerve and terminate in the descending nucleus. Subsequent connections are the same as those described above. Thus all the general somatic afferents of cranial nerves terminate in relation to the sensory trigeminal nuclei.

In cases of intractable lacerating pain from the face (trigeminal neuralgia, tic douloureux) the sensory root of the trigeminal nerve may be surgically sectioned or, since the pain fibers terminate in the subnucleus caudalis, the descending root may be cut low in the medulla, thus lessening the possibility of injury to other nerve roots. The spinothalamic tract is adjacent to the descending root in the medulla, and both may be involved in the same lesion. The result will be a loss of sense of pain and temperature change on the opposite side of the body since the secondary fibers of the spinothalamic tract cross in the spinal cord. There will be a loss of sense of pain and temperature change on the same side of the head due to the fact the primary fibers of the descending root are uncrossed.

7

Visceral Afferents and Referred Pain

Visceral afferents are divided into two functional components, general and special. The general conduct impulses arising from blood vessels and body cavity viscera, while the special are associated with the chemical senses of taste and smell. Olfactory pathways will be discussed in a later chapter.

The receptors in the general visceral afferent system are naked nerve endings, which respond to stretch and ischemia but not to cutting, burning, cold, or touch. Those fibers that convey pain from the viscera are directed into the spinal cord whereas those concerned primarily with reflex control of visceral organs enter the brain stem or sacral levels of the spinal cord. The cell bodies of the pain fibers are located in the dorsal root ganglia and are unipolar. The central process enters by way of the lateral division of the dorsal root, bifurcates, and terminates in the gray matter. Secondary neurons may effect reflex connections via internuncials with somatic neurons within the ventral horn and with preganglionic neurons associated with the autonomic nervous system. The pathway to higher centers for pain from the viscera is much more diffuse than that from the soma, and involves long and short fibers with numerous relays ascending bilaterally adjacent to the ventral horn. Upon reaching the brain stem the pathway continues via the reticular formation to the thalamus and hypothalamus. This pathway probably terminates principally in the nonspecific nuclei of the thalamus (centromedian, intralaminar, parafascicular, posterior) and constitutes part of the "slow" pain pathway as opposed to the "fast" pain pathway of the spinothalamic system. Visceral pain is characterized as being diffuse, persistent, and poorly localized.

General visceral afferents are carried by cranial nerves VII, IX, and X (Fig. 12). The fibers of X are distributed to receptors in the larynx, esophagus, and viscera in the thorax and abdomen. The fibers of IX arise from receptors in the oral pharynx and posterior one-third of the tongue. The few fibers of VII supply sensory innervation to a portion of the soft palate. All the cell bodies are unipolar and located in the geniculate ganglion of VII, petrosal ganglion of IX, and nodose ganglion of X. The central processes of these ganglion cells enter the solitary fasciculus which extends from the lower pons to the obex, where a few cross the midline and ascend a short distance in the contralateral solitary fasciculus. Surrounding this tract throughout its course is the solitary nucleus. The primary fibers coursing in the fasciculus solitarius terminate primarily in the caudal portion of the solitary nucleus. Secondary fibers arising from this nucleus effect reflex connections with various visceral motor nuclei (autonomic); others enter the reticular formation in which are located the vital centers controlling respiration and circulation; still others ascend via reticular pathways to higher visceral centers, particularly the hypothalamus. General visceral afferents concerned with the reflex control of pelvic visceral organs have their unipolar cell bodies located in the sacral dorsal root ganglia.

Taste buds are flask-shaped and are composed of supporting and neuroepithelial (taste) cells. The apex of the taste cell reaches the surface of the tongue by way of a pore. Extending from the apex of the taste cell into the pore are hair-like processes. Taste buds are found on the tongue in relation to the papillae, the palate, and epiglottis. The terminal end of

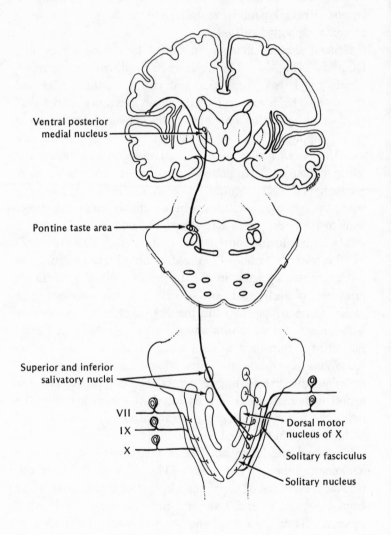

Ventral posterior
medial nucleus

Pontine taste area

Superior and inferior
salivatory nuclei

VII
IX
X

Dorsal motor
nucleus of X

Solitary fasciculus

Solitary nucleus

12. Visceral Afferent Pathways

sensory nerve fibers ramify on the surface of the taste cells. The facial nerve supplies the taste buds on the anterior two-thirds of the tongue; the glossopharyngeal on the posterior one-third; and the vagus on the epiglottis. The unipolar cell bodies are located in the geniculate ganglion of VII, petrosal ganglion of IX, and nodose ganglion of X (Fig. 12). The central processes descend in the solitary fasciculus and terminate, primarily in its cephalic portion. In some fish, which have numerous taste buds over their bodies, this nucleus is enlarged to the point where it fuses dorsally over the fourth ventricle with its fellow of the opposite side. It is absent in many birds and greatly reduced in mammals. Secondary fibers from the solitary nucleus terminate in visceral motor nuclei, which supply salivary glands. Others cross the midline and ascend to the upper pons where they terminate in the pontine taste area within and adjacent to the brachium conjunctivum. This area projects to the ventral posterior medial nucleus of the thalamus. En route some are given off to the hypothalamus. Tertiary fibers pass from the thalamus via the internal capsule and corona radiata to the primary gustatory cortex, which is located in the opercular portion of the post-central gyrus and probably the adjacent insular cortex.

Pain impulses arising from foci in the viscera may be interpreted as coming from a somatic area, a condition known as referred pain. Such pain is always referred from a visceral to a somatic area, both of which are supplied by the same sensory ganglion. There are several explanations why this phenomenon occurs. The viscera contain far fewer receptors per unit area than the soma, thus there is less awareness of the viscera. It has also been suggested that the incoming pain impulses from the viscera may sensitize a common neuronal pool from which both ascending visceral and somatic pathways arise. Some incoming visceral fibers may give off collaterals to cells in the dorsal horn which ultimately transmit impulses to

49

the spinothalamic system. Excitation of a common neuronal pool may explain the hyperesthesias frequently observed in the somatic zone along with sudomotor, vasomotor, and pilomotor changes and skeletal muscle spasms. All of these may contribute to the impression of pain arising from the soma. A cordotomy to relieve visceral pain must be bilateral and extend to the ventral horn gray, since the secondary visceral tracts ascend on both sides adjacent to the gray matter (fasciculus proprius).

8

Vestibular System

The receptors are neuroepithelial cells (hair cells) located in the cristae ampullaris of the semicircular canals and the maculae of the utricle and saccule of the inner ear (Fig. 13). The inner ear is in the petrous portion of the temporal bone. Although it is divided into cochlear and vestibular divisions, the structure is basically the same in that a membranous labyrinth is found within a bony enclosure, the osseous labyrinth. Otic fluid is present within the membranous labyrinth, and periotic in the osseous. The membranous portion of the vestibular division is composed of three semicircular canals which communicate with a sac-like structure, the utricle. The utricle is connected via a duct with the saccule. The point of attachment to the utricle of one arm of each of the semicircular canals is enlarged, forming the ampullae. On the wall of each ampulla is a thickening called the crista ampullaris. The cristae contain tall supporting cells and hair cells. The hairs project into a gelatinous mass, the cupula, which fills the ampulla. A portion of the wall of the utricle and saccule is thickened, forming the maculae, which are composed of supporting and hair cells and covered by a thin gelatinous mass. Embedded in the gelatinous substance are small concretions, the otoliths. Movement of the otic fluid within the semicircular canals displaces the cupula, stimulating the hair cells. In the maculae, gravity acts upon the otoliths, drawing them against or away from the hairs of the

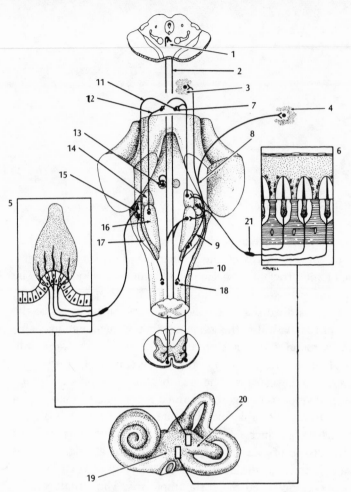

13. Vestibular System

1. Oculomotor nucleus 2. Medial longitudinal fasciculus 3. Nodulus 4. Flocculus 5. Crista 6. Macula 7. Nucleus fastigii 8. Ascending root of vestibular nerve 9. Descending root of vestibular nerve 10. Lateral vestibulospinal tract 11. Indirect fastigiobulbar tract 12. Direct fastigiobulbar tract 13. Abducens nucleus 14. Superior vestibular nucleus 15. Lateral vestibular nucleus 16. Medial vestibular nucleus 17. Descending vestibular nucleus 18. Reticular formation 19. Vestibule 20. Ampulla 21. Vestibular ganglion

sensory cells. Therefore, the cristae are the dynamic receptors which are stimulated by angular acceleration or deceleration and the maculae static receptors which indicate the position of the head. The sensory hairs of the receptor cells are stereocilia which are modified microvilli (40 to 100 per cell) and one peripheral kinocilium. Deviation of the stereocilia in the direction of the kinocilium increases the firing rate of the sensory cell whereas deviation in the opposite direction decreases the rate of firing.

The vestibular ganglion is located at the depths of the internal auditory meatus. The cells of this ganglion are bipolar. The peripheral processes terminate on the hair cells. The central processes pass in through the internal auditory meatus in company with the cochlear division of VIII and enter the brain stem at the junction of the pons and medulla. The vestibular division courses ventral and medial to the restiform body and bifurcates into ascending and descending roots. The fibers of the descending portion terminate on cells located in the lateral, medial, and spinal (descending) vestibular nuclei of the same side. The fibers of the ascending root terminate in the superior and medial vestibular nuclei and the cortex of the uvula, nodulus, and flocculus of the cerebellum. The portion of the ascending root that enters the cerebellum is a component of the juxtarestiform body. It should be pointed out that not all areas of the vestibular nuclei receive terminals from the vestibular nerve. Furthermore, specific portions of the labyrinth project to specific areas of the nuclei. However, it is beyond the scope of this book to discuss the complex organization of the vestibular nuclei.

A pathway to the cerebral cortex for the vestibular system no doubt exists, but the exact course has not been conclusively demonstrated. A vestibular cortical area has been identified in the temporal lobe adjacent to the primary auditory cortex in some animals. A second area in the face region of the postcentral gyrus has also been implicated. A few fibers from the vestibular nuclei to the ventral posterior lateral nucleus of the thalamus have been found. However, the bulk of the fibers from the vestibular nuclei to the thalamus must involve further relays. One nucleus thought to be involved is the interstitial nucleus of Cajal which is ventral to the oculomotor nucleus.

The vestibular system is primarily concerned with the reflex maintenance of the body and its parts in relation to space. To serve this function connections are made to the extrinsic muscles of the eye, the muscles of the neck, trunk, and extremities in that order of importance. Fibers arising from the vestibular nuclei ascend and descend on both sides in the medial longitudinal fasciculus. This tract extends in a dorsomedial position from upper midbrain levels to the cervical cord, where it is found in the ventral funiculus. In the spinal cord it is frequently referred to as the medial vestibulospinal tract. Ascending fibers of the medial longitudinal fasciculus terminate in the abducens, trochlear, and oculomotor nuclei, whose axons innervate the extraocular muscles.

Descending fibers in the medial longitudinal fasciculus enter the spinal cord and terminate on internuncial neurons in laminae VII and VIII. Axons from these neurons end on the ventral horn cells. By this connection the muscles of the neck and upper extremities are brought under vestibular reflex control. Another descending system of fibers arises from the lateral vestibular nucleus. It courses in the ventral and lateral funiculi and is known as the lateral vestibulospinal tract. These fibers terminate in the same laminae at all levels of the spinal cord. This brings the musculature of the trunk and extremities under vestibular control.

Other important projections of the vestibular nuclei are to the reticular formation and cerebellum. In addition to direct fibers from the vestibular nerve, the cerebellum receives vestibular impulses relayed by the vestibular nuclei. These fibers also enter the cerebellum by way of the juxtarestiform body and terminate in the nucleus fastigii and cortex of the flocculus, nodulus, and uvula of both sides. These areas are phylogenetically the oldest portions of the cerebellum and develop as a direct outgrowth of the vestibular nuclei. This portion of the cerebellum is vestibular in function and plays an important role in maintenance of equilibrium. The nucleus fastigii and cortical areas cited above as well as other areas of the vermis project to the vestibular nuclei and brain-stem reticular formation of the same side by way of the juxtarestiform body. This is known as the direct fastigiobulbar tract. Some fibers from the nucleus fastigii decussate in the cerebellar commissure, loop over the brachium conjunctivum, and exit with the juxtarestiform body to end in the opposite vestibular and reticular nuclei. This bundle is known as the uncinate fasciculus. Still others cross in the cerebellum and exit with the brachium conjunctivum, ending on cells in the mid-brain tegmentum and thalamus. These fibers constitute the ascending limb of the uncinate fasciculus.

Since the vestibular system is concerned with equilibrium, destructive lesions will result in impaired postural adjustments. If unilateral, the eyes, head, and body will turn to the affected side, and there will be vertigo and a tendency to fall to the side of the lesion. Nystagmus, a condition characterized by a slow movement of the eyes in one direction followed by a rapid return, is also present in involvement of any portion of the vestibular system. Irritative lesions result in forced movements, falling, nystagmus, vertigo (dizziness), and visceral disturbances (vomiting, sweating, etc.). The visceral disturbance is due to a discharge of the vestibular system into the reticular formation, which in turn is connected with various visceral motor nuclei. A good example of an irritative lesion is motion sickness.

9

Cochlear System

The cochlea is a spirally wound tube consisting of two and one-half turns around a central bony core, the modiolus (Fig. 14). The osseous labyrinth is divided into two canals, the scala vestibuli and scala tympani. The membranous labyrinth, or cochlear duct, is triangular and located between the scalae, and therefore sometimes referred to as the scala media: it is separated from the scala tympani by the basilar membrane and from the scala vestibuli by the vestibular membrane. The scalae, which are filled with periotic fluid, communicate with each other at the apex of the cochlea through a passage called the helicotrema. The cochlear duct contains otic fluid.

The hair cells located in the organ of Corti constitute the receptors of the cochlear system (Fig. 14). They are separated into a single row of inner hair cells and three parallel rows of outer hair cells by the tunnel of Corti. The apex of each hair cell contains stereocilia. The organ of Corti rests upon the basilar membrane and the hair cells are in contact with a firm fibrillar structure, the tectorial membrane. Pressure waves are set up in the periotic fluid of the scalae by movements of the foot plate of the stapes in the oval window. This results in vibration of the basilar membrane and stimulation of the hair cells via their contact with the tectorial membrane. Localization occurs in the organ of Corti in that the receptors at the apex are stimulated by low frequency sounds and at the base by high frequencies.

56

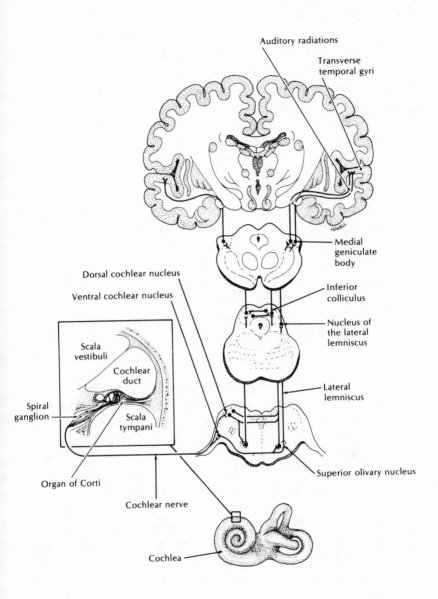

Auditory radiations

Transverse temporal gyri

Medial geniculate body

Dorsal cochlear nucleus

Ventral cochlear nucleus

Inferior colliculus

Nucleus of the lateral lemniscus

Scala vestibuli

Cochlear duct

Spiral ganglion

Scala tympani

Lateral lemniscus

Organ of Corti

Superior olivary nucleus

Cochlear nerve

Cochlea

14. Cochlear Pathways

The cell body of the primary neuron of the auditory pathway is located in the cochlear ganglion (spiral), which is found in the modiolus. The cell bodies are bipolar, with the peripheral processes terminating in relation to the hair cells of the organ of Corti. The vast majority of the fibers terminate in relation to the inner hair cells. Consequently, the inner hair cells are supplied with many more terminals than the outer. In addition to afferent fibers to the organ of Corti, there is a rich supply of efferent fibers that end on the hair cells. These fibers arise from the superior olivary nucleus and course in the olivocochlear bundle to the inner ear.

The central processes of spiral ganglion cells accompany the vestibular portion of the eighth nerve through the internal auditory meatus to enter the brain stem at the junction of the pons and medulla. These fibers pass dorsal to the restiform body, bifurcate, and terminate in the dorsal and ventral cochlear nuclei. The dorsal nucleus forms an eminence on the dorsolateral surface of the restiform body, whereas the ventral nucleus is located lateral to the restiform body.

Secondary fibers leave the cochlear nuclei in three striae (dorsal, intermediate, ventral) which traverse the upper medulla and pons and cross the midline. The fibers of the ventral stria cross through the ascending fibers of the medial lemniscus. The point at which the ventral stria and medial lemniscus intermingle is called the trapezoid body. Many of the fibers of the three striae terminate in relation to cells in the superior olivary nucleus, accessory superior olivary nucleus, and the nucleus of the trapezoid body of both sides. Others ascend in the contralateral lateral lemniscus, which at this point includes the spinothalamic tracts. Groups of neurons are found scattered within the lateral lemniscus in the upper pons. These are the nuclei of the lateral lemniscus and constitute nuclei of termination for some of the fibers in this lemniscus. The remaining fibers of the lateral lemniscus continue to the inferior colliculus of the midbrain, where virtually all terminate. It is possible that a few may bypass this nucleus to terminate in the medial geniculate body of the thalamus. Fibers arising from the nucleus of the inferior colliculus ascend through the brachium of the inferior colliculus (central acoustic tract) and terminate in the medial geniculate body. Fibers from the medial geniculate body course in the sublenticular portion (auditory radiations) of the internal capsule to terminate in the primary auditory cortex (superior and transverse temporal gyri). Some fibers of the ascending pathway are uncrossed. Furthermore, there are considerable cross connections, particularly between the inferior colliculi and nuclei of the lateral lemniscus.

Descending pathways are also present in the auditory system. The auditory cortex gives rise to fibers which terminate in the medial geniculate body and the inferior colliculus. The latter in turn sends fibers to the superior olivary nucleus and the cochlear nuclei. As pointed out previously, the superior olivary nucleus gives rise to the olivocochlear bundle which terminates on the hair cells of the organ of Corti.

The nuclei found throughout the course of the auditory pathway (nucleus of the trapezoid body, superior olivary nucleus, accessory superior olivary nucleus, nucleus of the lateral lemniscus, nucleus of the inferior colliculus) serve as relay nuclei in the pathway and as reflex centers. Consequently the fibers arising from these nuclei will project forward in the auditory pathway, e.g. lateral lemniscus. Other connections of these nuclei are made with reticular nuclei, and by way of the medial longitudinal fasciculus to various motor nuclei of cranial nerves and in the intermediate gray of the spinal cord. The latter project to the ventral horn cells. These reflex connections form the basis for reflex movements of the eyes, head, and trunk in response to sound.

In addition to serving as reflex centers and relay stations, the various nuclei in the auditory pathway which are under the in-

59

fluence of both ascending and descending fibers are involved in more complex functions. The ability to discriminate frequencies is probably carried out at levels below the medial geniculate body and is not dependent on that nucleus or the cortex. Tonotopic localization is present in the organ of Corti as well as throughout the central pathway. No doubt, central mechanisms play an important role in screening out unwanted auditory signals so that a high degree of discrimination is possible.

Localization of sound in space is also a function of the several nuclei as well as the cortex. However, the ability is greatly reduced following deafness in one ear. Intensity discrimination is dependent on both the organ of Corti and the various nuclei. The cortex does not seem to play an important role. On the other hand, the cortex is important in discriminating patterns of sound such as those occurring in speech. This may be related to the necessity of short-term memory in speech.

Unilateral lesions that completely destroy the receptors, cochlear nerve, or cochlear nuclei will cause total deafness in that ear. Central unilateral lesions (cortex, medial geniculate body, lateral lemniscus) result in impaired hearing in both ears, but more marked on the opposite side. Isolated lesions of specific parts of the organ of Corti may result in deafness to a specific pitch or tone. Conduction deafness results from involvement of those organs conducting sound waves to the receptors, e.g. ear ossicles, but bone conduction is not impaired in these cases, i.e. a tuning fork placed on the skull can be heard. Irritative lesions result in hissing and roaring sounds. These usually precede a destructive lesion.

10

Visual System

The retina, which contains the light receptors, is the innermost layer of the eye. Embryologically, it is formed from an evagination of the diencephalon. Three basic types of nerve cells are present in the retina: rod and cone cells, bipolar cells, and ganglion cells (Fig. 15). The outermost are the rod and cone cells, whose dendrites are modified to form rods and cones. The rods, numbering over 100 million, are slender elongated modifications of the dendritic end. The cones, of which there are about 7 million, are shorter and thicker. In the center of the retina is a circular yellowish spot, the macula lutea, which is depressed in the middle, forming the fovea centralis. The fovea contains only cones and is devoid of any other retinal layer, except for the pigmented layer. The cones decrease in number toward the periphery, whereas the rods increase. Outside the rods and cones is a layer of pigmented cells. The pigment migrates with varying degrees of illumination, increasing in amount between the receptors in bright light.

Each rod and cone consists of an outer segment, a connecting stalk, and an inner segment. The outer segment is composed of a series of discs stacked one on another. In the rods the discs contain rhodopsin and are free in that they are not continuous with the outer membrane of the rod. The discs are continuously cast off at the apex and reformed at the base from rhodopsin synthesized in the inner segment. The discarded discs are dis-

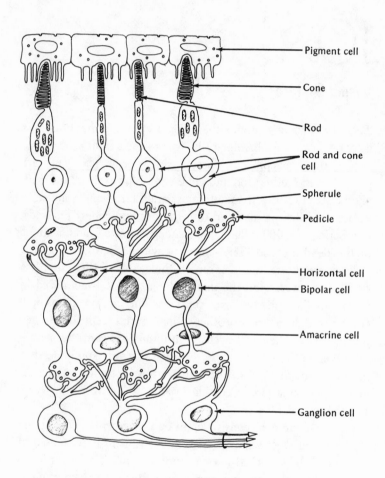

Pigment cell

Cone

Rod

Rod and cone cell

Spherule

Pedicle

Horizontal cell

Bipolar cell

Amacrine cell

Ganglion cell

15. Histology of the Retina

62

posed of by the pigment cells. The discs within the cones are continuous with the outer membrane and contain one of three photosensitive pigments; they are thus referred to as blue, green, or red cones. The connecting stalk of the rods and cones is narrow and contains a cilium. The inner segment contains mitochondria and the Golgi apparatus and is the site of synthesis of the photoreceptor pigment. Extending from the end of the cell opposite to the rod is a process which ends as a bulbous enlargement, the spherule. In the cone this ending is flattened, forming a pedicle.

Each pedicle and spherule has numerous synapses with bipolar and horizontal cells. Bipolar cells transmit in the vertical direction whereas the horizontal cells allow for the lateral spread of excitation in the retina. The ganglion cells located internal to the bipolar cells are in synaptic contact with them as well as amacrine cells. The latter are devoid of axons and, like the horizontal cells, have processes which extend laterally. The axons of ganglion cells form a layer of fibers adjacent to the vitreous body as they converge on the optic disc where they exit as the optic nerve. The optic disc is devoid of other retinal elements and is thus the blind spot. Filling in the interstices between the various cells and processes of the retina are Müller's cells. They also form two membranes: one at the level of the rods and cones and the other between the vitreous body and optic nerve fibers.

As a result of the arrangement of cells, fibers, and synaptic areas, ten retinal layers can be recognized. The outermost is the layer of pigment cells (1). Adjacent to this are the rods and cones (2), followed by the outer limiting membrane (3). The outer nuclear layer (4) consists of the cell bodies of the rod and cone cells. The synaptic zone between the rod and cone cells and bipolar and horizontal neurons is the outer plexiform layer (5). Adjacent to this is the inner nuclear layer (6), which consists largely of bipolar cells. The inner plexiform layer (7) is the synaptic zone between bipolar and amacrine neurons and ganglion cells. The multipolar neurons form the ganglionic cell layer (8), and their axons form the layer of optic nerve fibers (9). Finally, the inner limiting membrane (10) separates the retina from the vitreous body. Therefore, to reach the rods and cones, light must penetrate all retinal layers except the pigmented layer. However, at the fovea centralis the other retinal layers are absent.

The optic nerve, like the retina, is an extension of the central nervous system and is, therefore, not a true nerve. It courses back through the optic foramen to the optic chiasma, where half the fibers decussate (Fig. 16). From the optic chiasma the fibers are known as the optic tract, which passes back to enter the diencephalon, where most of the fibers terminate in the lateral geniculate body. The axons of the cells in the lateral geniculate body give rise to the optic radiations. These course in the retrolenticular portion of the internal capsule and then in the lateral wall of the temporal horn of the lateral ventricle to the calcarine cortex (cuneus and lingual gyri).

There is a topographical relationship between specific quadrants of the retina and specific points along the optic pathway. Fibers from the medial half of the retina and medial half of the macula course in the medial half of the optic nerve and cross in the optic chiasma to the medial half of the opposite optic tract. Fibers from the macula occupy the center of the optic nerve and tract. Fibers from the lateral half of the retina and lateral half of the macula course in the lateral half of the optic nerve and optic tract of the same side. They do not cross in the optic chiasma. Fibers from the macula terminate in the posterior superior portion of the lateral geniculate body. Fibers from the lower quadrants of the retina end in the lateral portion of the lateral geniculate body, whereas those from the upper quadrants terminate medially. Fibers of the optic radiations conveying impulses from the upper quadrants of the retina course in the superior part of the radiations and terminate in the cuneus, the superior

64

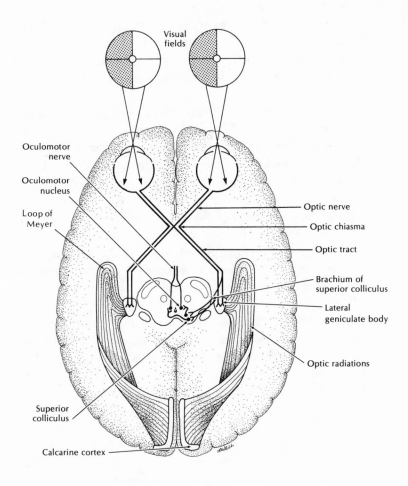

Visual fields

Oculomotor nerve

Oculomotor nucleus

Loop of Meyer

Optic nerve

Optic chiasma

Optic tract

Brachium of superior colliculus

Lateral geniculate body

Optic radiations

Superior colliculus

Calcarine cortex

16. Visual Pathways

65

part of the calcarine cortex. The inferior fibers of the radiations pass forward in the temporal lobe as the loop of Meyer before turning back to the occipital lobe. They convey impulses from the lower quadrants of the retina to the lingual gyrus, the inferior part of the calcarine cortex. Fibers of the radiations conveying impulses from the macula occupy an intermediate position, and terminate in the posterior portion of the calcarine cortex.

It must be remembered that the visual fields and retinal quadrants are reversed. Light from below a horizontal plane, passing through the center of the pupil, falls on the upper retinal quadrants. Light from above this plane falls on the lower retinal quadrants. Light from the right falls on the nasal retina of the right eye and temporal retina of the left eye. Light from the left falls on the nasal retina of the left eye and temporal retina of the right eye. Therefore, since the fibers from the nasal retina cross in the optic chiasma, the left visual field is represented in the right optic tract, lateral geniculate body, optic radiations, and calcarine cortex. The right visual field is represented in the left optic tract, etc.

A few fibers of the optic tract bypass the lateral geniculate body to enter the brachium of the superior colliculus and terminate in the superior colliculus and pretectal region. These fibers are joined by a few arising from the lateral geniculate body. Fibers from the superior colliculus and pretectal region terminate in the parasympathetic portion of the third nerve nucleus (Edinger-Westphal). This is the anatomical basis for the pupillary constriction reflex to light. From the pretectal region and superior colliculus, fibers descend via the medial longitudinal fasciculus, tectospinal tract, and by short relays through the reticular formation, to the intermediolateral cell column of the upper thoracic segments. This is the basis for the sympathetic pupillary dilator reflex to light. The accommodation reflex, which includes pupillary constriction, thickening of the lens, and

66

convergence of the eyes, involves a pathway through the cerebral cortex. There are other reflexes to light, involving reflex movement of the eyes, head, etc., which have diffuse pathways but which apparently arise from the pretectal region and superior colliculus. Some fibers cross in the posterior commissure, resulting in crossed reflexes.

It should be remembered that the superior colliculus and pretectal region have connections with other areas of the central nervous system. These include the cortex, lateral geniculate body, inferior colliculus, substantia nigra, reticular formation, cerebellum, vestibular nuclei, and spinal cord. Therefore, these areas are more than simple reflex centers. For example, they are important in tracking movements, i.e. orientation of the eyes, head, and body in relation to auditory and visual stimuli.

A complete lesion of the optic nerve will result in total blindness in that eye. If the optic tract is severed, however, the defect will be in the opposite visual field since fibers from the nasal retina cross. This is known as homonymous hemianopsia. The same condition results from the total destruction of the lateral geniculate body, optic radiations, or visual cortex. A lesion of the optic chiasma interrupting only the decussating fibers results in bitemporal hemianopsia, i.e. the temporal portion of the visual field of each eye is affected. Destruction of the superior portion of the optic radiations or cuneus results in opposite lower quadrantic defects, whereas involvement of the lower radiations or lingual gyrus gives rise to opposite upper quadrantic defects. Lesions of the pretectal region and/or superior colliculus abolish reflexes to light but do not impair visual acuity. If the posterior commissure is involved, crossed reflexes are absent.

11

Dorsal Thalamus

The diencephalon is divided into four divisions: epithalamus, hypothalamus, subthalamus, and dorsal thalamus. The epithalamus has strong connections with the olfactory system and will be discussed in Chapter 18. The hypothalamus is associated with basic vegetative functions and will be covered under the autonomic nervous system. The subthalamus is related to the extrapyramidal system. The dorsal thalamus is composed of a number of nuclei, most of which have numerous subdivisions. It is not within the scope of this work to discuss exhaustively all the nuclei—only the major nuclear groups will be covered.

The internal medullary lamina of the dorsal thalamus separates the nuclei into two major groups: the medial-anterior group and lateral-ventral group (Fig. 17). The lamina is composed of myelinated fibers entering or leaving the adjacent thalamic nuclei. The external medullary lamina is medial to the internal capsule. Its fibers interconnect the thalamic nuclei with the cerebral cortex.

The anterior nucleus has extensive reciprocal connections with the gyrus cinguli, but its principal afferent tract is the mammillothalamic fasciculus. Some fibers of the fornix also end in this nucleus. Since the gyrus cinguli is a portion of the limbic lobe, which is concerned with autonomic functions and emotional tone, the anterior nucleus plays an important role in these activities.

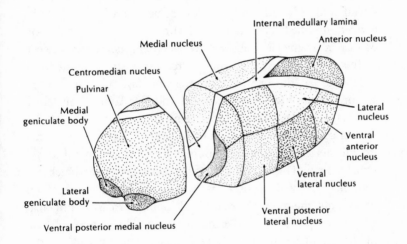

Internal medullary lamina

Medial nucleus

Anterior nucleus

Centromedian nucleus

Pulvinar

Medial
geniculate body

Lateral
nucleus

Ventral
anterior
nucleus

Lateral
geniculate body

Ventral
lateral nucleus

Ventral posterior medial nucleus

Ventral posterior
lateral nucleus

17. Dorsal Thalamus

69

The medial (dorsomedial) nucleus has extensive reciprocal connections with the prefrontal lobes, and also receives numerous fibers from the amygdala, the ventral posterior nucleus of the thalamus, and probably the hypothalamus. The prefrontal lobes are related to personality, ideation, and affective tone, i.e. feeling of well being. These states are readily altered by external and internal sensations. The medial nucleus plays a role in these functions by way of its connections with the amygdala, hypothalamus, and ventral posterior nucleus. The hypothalamus receives extensive visceral afferents, whereas the ventral posterior nucleus is associated with the main somatic sensory pathways.

The ventral nucleus is divisible into three segments: anterior, lateral, and posterior; the posterior segment can further be subdivided into medial and lateral. All three portions are important cortical relay nuclei which receive ascending fibers and project to the cortex. The ventral anterior receives a strong input from the globus pallidus by way of the thalamic fasciculus. It also has an input from the substantia nigra and intralaminar nuclei of the thalamus. Its efferent projections are to wide areas of the frontal cortex, including the motor areas. It seems to be functionally related to the intralaminar nuclei and the extrapyramidal system. The ventral lateral nucleus receives the brachium conjunctivum which arises in the cerebellum. It also receives fibers from the globus pallidus and motor cortex. Its principal efferent projection is to the motor cortex. The trigeminal lemniscus terminates in the ventral posterior medial nucleus and the medial lemniscus and spinothalamic tracts end in the ventral posterior lateral. Both these nuclei send fibers to the postcentral gyrus.

The strongest connections of the lateral nucleus are with the posterior portion of the parietal lobe and pass in both directions. The lateral nucleus also is related to adjacent thalamic nuclei. Since the posterior parietal lobe is an important association area concerned with interpreting and integrating various sensory modalities, the lateral nucleus plays a role in reinforcing these functions.

The pulvinar and medial and lateral geniculate bodies may also be included in the lateral and ventral group of thalamic nuclei. The two geniculate bodies are primarily cortical relay nuclei. The medial geniculate body receives the brachium of the inferior colliculus and projects as auditory radiations to the primary auditory cortex. The optic tract terminates in the lateral geniculate body, which gives rise to the optic radiations terminating in the primary visual cortex.

The pulvinar is associated with the posterior parietal, lateral occipital, and posterior temporal cortices. The connections are two-way. These cortical areas are association centers, and thus the pulvinar is related to these functions. The pulvinar has connections with other thalamic nuclei, particularly the ventral posterior and the geniculate bodies.

The dorsal thalamus contains, in addition, four poorly defined nuclear groups: reticular, intralaminar, posterior, and midline. The reticular nuclei, which are scattered patches of cells in the external medullary lamina, receive fibers from wide areas of the cortex and most thalamic nuclei. They project to the thalamic nuclei and as far caudal as the mesencephalon. They may be concerned with integrating thalamic activity and corticothalamic impulses. The intralaminar nuclei are located within the internal medullary lamina. One portion is well developed, forming the discrete centromedian nucleus. Another important nucleus of this group is the parafascicular. The intralaminar nuclei receive numerous fibers from the reticular formation. Some spinothalamic fibers also terminate there. They may also receive fibers from the cortex and globus pallidus. They project to the putamen and other thalamic nuclei, particularly the ventral anterior. They may also send some fibers to the cortex. They appear to be a part of the ascending activating system and to play a role in thalamic integration. The midline nuclei are gray masses in the wall of the third ventricle and include the massa intermedia, which bridges the ventricle. They are associated with the hypothalamus and basal ganglia and are related to basic vegetative functions. The posterior complex is an ill-defined group of nuclei at the mesodiencephalic junction. These nuclei receive fibers from the spinothalamic tract as well as the reticular formation. Cortical connections are made with the insular and auditory cortex. They may be concerned with central pain mechanisms.

Although a clear distinction cannot be made, it is convenient to speak of specific and nonspecific nuclei. The former are sometimes referred to as cortically dependent, since they have extensive connections with the cortex. These include the cortical relay nuclei whose primary input is from ascending pathways and whose output is to the cortex (geniculate bodies, ventral posterior, ventral lateral, and anterior nuclei). The specific cortical association nuclei do not have connections with ascending systems but are reciprocally related to other thalamic nuclei as well as to the cortex (pulvinar, lateral, and medial nuclei). The nonspecific nuclei have, at best, very few connections with the cortex but are associated with subcortical structures (reticular, midline, posterior, and intralaminar nuclei). The ventral anterior nucleus seems to have characteristics of both specific and nonspecific nuclei.

Because of the multiplicity of functions of the dorsal thalamus a wide variety of signs and symptoms may result from destructive lesions. Intellectual deterioration may occur with involvement of the lateral nucleus and pulvinar. Personality changes occur with the destruction of the medial nucleus. If the lesion encroaches on the ventral posterior nucleus there is contralateral loss of position sense and touch discrimination. Ataxia, an awkward gait, is present due to loss of knowledge of the position of the limbs. Awareness of pain and of temperature persist but are poorly localized; the feeling of pain may be greatly exaggerated. Involvement of the lateral geniculate body gives rise to homonymous hemianopsia.

12

Lower Motor Neurons and General
Aspects of Motor Systems

Nuclei giving rise to fibers innervating skeletal muscle derived from myotomes are referred to as general somatic efferent. Special visceral efferent fibers supply skeletal muscles of branchial arch origin. General visceral efferents innervate the viscera and will be discussed in the chapter on the autonomic nervous system. The general somatic efferent column of cells is adjacent to the midline directly under the cerebral aqueduct, fourth ventricle, and ventrolateral to the central canal. It is represented in the midbrain by the oculomotor nucleus, which innervates the levator palpebrae superioris, inferior oblique, and superior, medial, and inferior rectus muscles of the eye (Fig. 18). The trochlear nucleus is in the lower midbrain. It supplies only the superior oblique muscle of the eye. The abducens nucleus, which innervates the lateral rectus, is located in the lower pons. The hypoglossal nucleus, whose fibers supply the intrinsic muscles of the tongue and the styloglossus, hyoglossus, and genioglossus, is found throughout a considerable extent of the medulla. The general somatic efferent column in the spinal cord is represented by the large alpha motor neurons in lamina IX of the ventral horn. They innervate the muscles of the trunk and extremities. Most of the small neurons in lamina IX are gamma efferents. However, some of them may be Renshaw cells. These receive collaterals

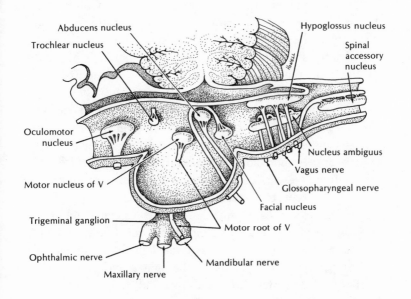

Abducens nucleus

Trochlear nucleus

Hypoglossus nucleus

Spinal accessory nucleus

Oculomotor nucleus

Nucleus ambiguus

Vagus nerve

Motor nucleus of V

Glossopharyngeal nerve

Trigeminal ganglion

Facial nucleus

Ophthalmic nerve

Motor root of V

Maxillary nerve

Mandibular nerve

18. Lower Motor Nuclei

from the exiting alpha fibers which in turn synapse on the motor neuron completing an inhibitory circuit. The fibers of all general somatic efferent nuclei exit ventrally except those of the trochlear, which, after decussating, emerge caudal to the inferior colliculus on the dorsal aspect of the brain stem.

The special visceral efferent column of cells is ventral and lateral to the general somatic efferent group. Fibers arising from these nuclei course for a variable distance dorsally and medially, turn sharply back, forming a loop, and exit laterally. The motor nucleus of the trigeminal nerve is located in the upper pons and supplies the muscles of mastication, the mylohyoid, anterior belly of the digastric, tensor tympani, and tensor veli palatini. These muscles come from the first branchial arch. The facial nucleus, whose fibers innervate the facial muscles, the stylohyoid, stapedius, and posterior belly of the digastric, is in the lower pons. These muscles are derived from the second branchial arch. The nucleus ambiguus consists of a thin column of cells extending throughout most of the medulla. Fibers from the cephalic portion supply the stylopharyngeus muscle by way of the glossopharyngeal nerve. This muscle arises embryologically from the third branchial arch. Fibers from the caudal portion of the nucleus ambiguus join the vagus nerve to innervate the intrinsic muscles of the larynx and the striated muscles of the pharynx and upper esophagus. These muscles develop from the fourth and fifth arches. The accessory nucleus is located in the lower medulla and upper cervical segments of the spinal cord and supplies portions of the sternocleidomastoid and trapezius muscles, which are derived in part from the caudal portion of the branchial arch system.

Each motor fiber terminates in relation to a motor end plate found on the muscle fiber (Fig. 19). The surface of the muscle fiber covered with sarcolemma is thrown into folds, forming clefts in between the elevations. The nerve fiber as

76

it approaches the muscle divides into a variable number of branches and loses its myelin sheath. The terminal end of the nerve fiber retains its neurilemma and sends branches into the clefts on the muscle fiber. Surrounding the motor end plate in the adjacent sarcoplasm is a concentration of nuclei. The nerve fiber terminals contain mitochondria and synaptic vesicles which in turn contain the transmitter substance acetylcholine. A single efferent neuron plus the muscle fibers it innervates constitute a motor unit. The ratio of muscle fibers to the motor neuron becomes progressively smaller with the degree to which the muscles are capable of carrying out fine discrete movements.

Cells within the motor nuclei are frequently referred to as lower motor neurons or the final common path. All motor systems, from reflex mechanisms to voluntary motor activity, must converge on these neurons for their influences to reach the effectors. Descending tracts from higher centers (supranuclear or upper motor neurons) or afferent fibers of peripheral nerves do not terminate, with few exceptions, directly upon the lower motor neuron (Fig. 19). Instead they end in relation to the intermediate gray and the base of the dorsal horn in the spinal cord, and in the reticular formation surrounding the motor nuclei in the brain stem. Cells in these areas synapse with the motor neurons. The exceptions to the general rule include some of the fibers of the pyramidal tract (the voluntary motor system) and a few sensory fibers of peripheral nerves mediating the myotatic reflex.

Since all motor systems and afferents from peripheral receptors converge on the intermediate gray and reticular formation, these areas become important correlation and integration centers. All the systems above play an important role in motor activity and are in delicate balance with each other since there are numerous feedback circuits between the higher centers. In any motor act they all send information to the

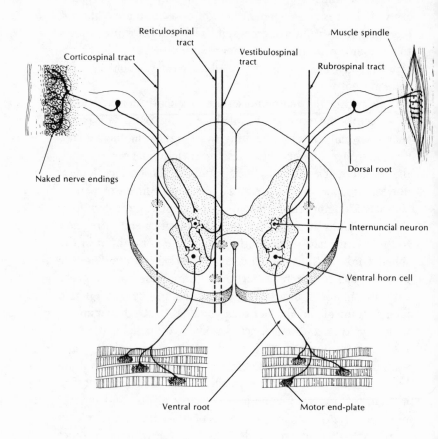

Reticulospinal tract

Muscle spindle

Corticospinal tract

Vestibulospinal tract

Rubrospinal tract

Naked nerve endings

Dorsal root

Internuncial neuron

Ventral horn cell

Ventral root

Motor end-plate

19. Termination of Motor Pathways

reticular formation and intermediate gray, which correlates this information and projects the final pattern on the lower motor neurons. These in turn conduct the impulses to the appropriate effectors.

If the lower motor neurons are destroyed, such as in lesions of the peripheral nerves or motor nuclei, total paralysis of the muscles supplied by these cells results. No impulses can reach the muscles, which are thus completely flaccid. Reflexes are absent. If the lesion involves upper motor neurons, the muscles are not completely paralyzed since the lower motor neurons are intact and some impulses still reach the muscles. However, since all motor centers play a role in motor activity, destruction of one destroys the delicate balance between them, and the normal pattern of motor activity is altered. The affected muscles still exhibit some tone, but they may be hypertonic (spasticity or rigidity) or hypotonic depending on the location of the lesion; and there may be hyper- or hyporeflexia. Other symptoms present may be the paralysis of some movements and presence of abnormal movements.

13

Cerebellum

The cerebellum is located dorsal to the medulla and pons and is overlapped by the occipital lobes of the cerebral hemispheres. Two cerebellar hemispheres can be recognized, separated by a midline vermis. The cerebellum can be divided into numerous lobules but for the purpose of this work only three major lobes will be recognized. The first fissure to appear is the uvulonodular and its hemispheric extension, the posterolateral fissure. Posterior to these fissures is the flocculonodular lobe. The nodulus is vermis, and the flocculi hemispheric. On the superior surface of the cerebellum is found the primary fissure. The anterior lobe is forward to this. The posterior lobe, composing the largest portion of the cerebellum, is located between the primary and uvulonodular fissures. The flocculonodular lobe is phylogenetically the oldest portion of the cerebellum and is associated with the vestibular system. It is referred to as archicerebellum. The anterior lobe along with the uvula and pyramis in the posterior vermal portion of the posterior lobe constitute the paleocerebellum. The remainder of the posterior lobe makes up the neocerebellum, which develops in relation to the neocortex.

The surface of the cerebellum is thrown into numerous transverse folds known as folia. The cortex is located superficially (Fig. 21, p. 84). The central core of the cerebellum contains white matter, at the base of which are the deep cerebellar nuclei.

The structure of the cortex is uniform (Fig. 20). It consists of three layers which, from superficial to deep, are: molecular layer, Purkinje (ganglionic) cell layer, and granule cell layer. The molecular layer contains principally dendrites and axons of cells in the deep layers. It is thus an important synaptic zone. Present within this zone are a few neurons known as basket cells and stellate cells. The axons course at right angles to the long axis of the folia. Collaterals and terminals form basket-like synaptic endings around the Purkinje cells. The axons of stellate cells run transversely and synapse with dendrites of Purkinje cells. The Purkinje cells are large neurons forming a single layer deep to the molecular layer. They contain an apical dendrite which branches profusely in the molecular layer at right angles to the long axis of the folium. The axon arises from the base and terminates in the deep cerebellar nuclei. The granule layer contains a large number of small neurons, the granule cells. These neurons have many short dendrites and an axon which enters the molecular layer. The axon bifurcates and runs parallel with the long axis of the folium. It comes into synaptic contact with the dendrites of a large number of Purkinje cells, as well as with basket and stellate cells. Golgi cells are also found in the granular layer. Their axons end in complex glomeruli formed by the terminal ends of incoming fibers and dendrites of granule cells. The dendrites are in synaptic relation with axons of granule cells.

The afferent fibers to the cerebellar cortex terminate as either mossy or climbing fibers. The climbing fibers end in relation to the dendrites of the Purkinje cell. The mossy fibers end in a rosette within a glomerulus. Also entering the glomerulus are the dendrites of many granule cells and the axons of Golgi cells. The efferent neuron of the cortex is the Purkinje cell, which also sends collaterals to the Golgi cell. Numerous circuits through the cortex are possible, but they must finally converge on the Purkinje cell. There is a balance between

81

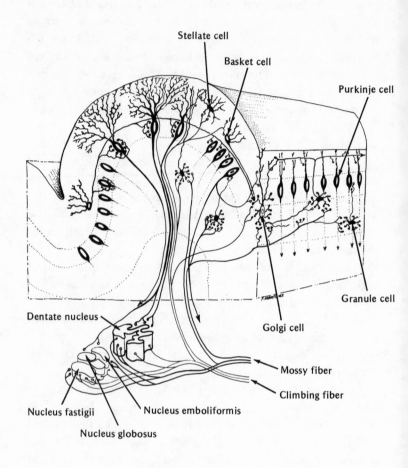

Stellate cell

Basket cell

Purkinje cell

Granule cell

Golgi cell

Dentate nucleus

Mossy fiber

Climbing fiber

Nucleus fastigii

Nucleus emboliformis

Nucleus globosus

20. Cerebellar Cortex

82

inhibition and excitation through the various circuits in the cortex. The climbing fiber excites the Purkinje cell. The mossy fiber is excitatory to the granule cell, which in turn also excites the Purkinje cell. The granule cell excites the stellate, basket, and Golgi cells. The stellate and basket cells inhibit the Purkinje cell, whereas the Golgi cell inhibits the granule cell. Finally, the Purkinje cell is inhibitory to the deep cerebellar nuclei.

The afferent fibers of the cerebellum traverse the three cerebellar peduncles (Fig. 21). The inferior cerebellar peduncle (restiform body) is entirely afferent with the exception of its medial portion, which is designated the juxtarestiform body. This was discussed in the chapter on the vestibular system. Other components of the inferior peduncle are: dorsal spinocerebellar tract, olivocerebellar fibers, trigeminocerebellar fibers, direct arcuate fibers, arcuocerebellar fibers, and a reticulocerebellar component. The dorsal spinocerebellar tract arises from the homolateral nucleus dorsalis in the thoracic cord. This nucleus receives terminals from the dorsal funiculus and constitutes a pathway to the cerebellum for exteroceptive and proprioceptive impulses from the lower half of the body. The dorsal spinocerebellar tract terminates in the vermis. The olivocerebellar fibers originate in the inferior olivary nucleus in the medulla, are entirely crossed, and terminate in most areas of the cerebellar cortex as climbing fibers. The inferior olivary nucleus receives fibers from two sources: spino-olivary tract and central tegmental fasciculus. The spino-olivary tract arises from the contralateral dorsal horn. The spino-olivocerebellar pathway may constitute another pathway to the cerebellum for touch and proprioception. The central tegmental fasciculus has a diffuse origin. Fibers to the inferior olive arise from the motor cortex, red nucleus, pretectal region, and superior colliculus as well as other scattered nuclei in the brain stem. It is apparent that the inferior olive serves as a point of convergence

83

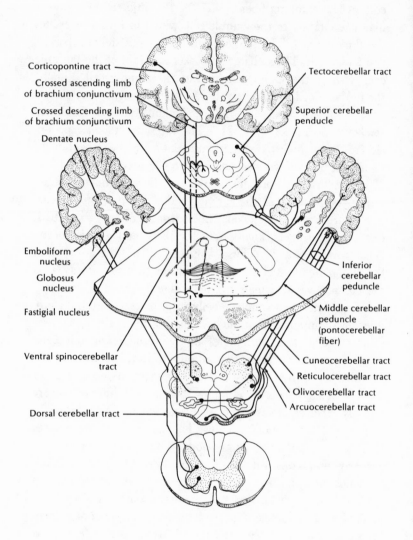

Corticopontine tract

Crossed ascending limb of brachium conjunctivum

Crossed descending limb of brachium conjunctivum

Dentate nucleus

Emboliform nucleus

Globosus nucleus

Fastigial nucleus

Ventral spinocerebellar tract

Dorsal cerebellar tract

Tectocerebellar tract

Superior cerebellar penducle

Inferior cerebellar peduncle

Middle cerebellar peduncle (pontocerebellar fiber)

Cuneocerebellar tract

Reticulocerebellar tract

Olivocerebellar tract

Arcuocerebellar tract

21. Cerebellar Connections

84

of impulses for areas serving a variety of functions and in turn influences the activity of almost all of the cerebellar cortex.

The trigeminocerebellar fibers arise from the subnuclei interpolaris and rostralis of the descending nucleus of V. They are both crossed and uncrossed and terminate in the vermis. This is the pathway for tactile impulses from the head to the cerebellum. Direct arcuate fibers arise from the homolateral external cuneate nucleus. They also terminate in the vermis. Since this nucleus receives terminals from the fasciculus cuneatus, the direct arcuate fibers are in the pathway from the proprioceptors and tactile receptors in the neck and upper extremities to the cerebellum. The arcuate nuclei are found in the medullary pyramid and are probably displaced pontine nuclei. They receive fibers from the homolateral motor cortex and are concerned with relating that area to the cerebellum. Arcuocerebellar fibers cross the midline and circle the periphery of the medulla as ventral external arcuate fibers. They end in the cerebellar hemispheres. Certain reticular nuclei project into the cerebellum from both sides, either directly or by way of the ventral external arcuate fibers. They terminate largely in the vermis and anterior lobe. Afferents to these nuclei arise from a variety of nuclei, however the largest input is from the cortex and spinal cord.

The middle cerebellar peduncle (brachium pontis) is likewise entirely afferent and contains one component, the pontocerebellar fibers. These are entirely crossed and arise from the pontine nuclei. They terminate in the neocerebellar cortex of the hemispheres. A large bundle of fibers, the corticopontine tract, arises from the motor cortex and descends uncrossed to terminate in the pontine nuclei. These two tracts form the corticopontocerebellar pathway, which is an important link between the motor areas of the neocortex and the neocerebellum.

The superior cerebellar peduncle (brachium conjunctivum) is mixed, the efferent component being the largest. It will be

85

discussed below. The ventral spinocerebellar tract arises from scattered cells of the dorsal and intermediate gray of the spinal cord of both sides. It ascends ventral to the dorsal tract, but in the medulla when the dorsal tract enters the inferior peduncle it continues to the upper pons, loops back, and enters the cerebellum with the superior peduncle to terminate in the vermis. It forms another pathway for exteroceptive and proprioceptive impulses from the lower half of the body to the cerebellum. The main sensory nucleus of the trigeminal nerve sends some fibers to the cerebellar vermis by way of the superior peduncle. This is another link between somatic receptors in the head and the cerebellum. The tectocerebellar tract arising from the superior and inferior colliculi convey visual and auditory impressions into the cerebellum by way of the superior peduncle.

Four pairs of nuclei can be recognized in the medullary core at the base of the cerebellum. They are, from medial to lateral: fastigial, globosus, emboliformis, and dentate. The connections of the nucleus fastigii with the flocculonodular lobe, vestibular nuclei, and reticular formation have been discussed in the chapter on the vestibular system. The globosus and emboliformis nuclei are small. A portion of the globosus is related to the vestibular system while the remainder, and the emboliformis nuclei, have the same connections as the dentate. The dentate is a large convoluted nucleus which receives fibers from the Purkinje cells of the cerebellar cortex. The dentate nucleus gives rise to a compact bundle of fibers, the superior cerebellar peduncle (brachium conjunctivum), which courses cephalically in the superior medullary velum. In the upper pons and lower midbrain the superior cerebellar peduncle turns ventral and medial to decussate with its fellow of the opposite side.

After crossing, a small bundle of fibers is given off which descends through the tegmentum of the midbrain and pons and reticular formation of the medulla. This is the crossed descending limb of the brachium conjunctivum. It terminates in relation to nuclear groups in the tegmentum and reticular formation.

The remaining fibers, constituting the crossed ascending limb of the brachium conjunctivum, course through and around the red nucleus. A number of the fibers terminate here and the remainder continue into the thalamus to end in the ventral lateral and centromedian nuclei. The former projects through the internal capsule to the motor areas of the cortex. The centromedian nucleus sends fibers into the basal ganglia. These connections complete feedback circuits between the cerebellum on the one hand and the motor cortex on the other.

Descending fibers from the red nucleus cross ventral to the red nucleus and descend as the rubrospinal tract in the lateral portion of the brain stem and lateral funiculus of the spinal cord, terminating in the intermediate gray. Other descending fibers contribute to the central tegmental fasciculus to end in the inferior olivary nucleus.

It is convenient to subdivide the cerebellum functionally as well as anatomically into the vestibulocerebellum, which corresponds closely to the flocculonodular lobe, the spinocerebellum (anterior lobe), and the pontocerebellum (posterior lobe). The vestibulocerebellum has its principal input from the vestibular nerve and nuclei and projects via the nucleus fastigii to the vestibular nuclei and reticular formation. This area controls posture and equilibrium. The spinocerebellum receives fibers from the spinal cord, e.g. spinocerebellar tracts, spino-olivocerebellar pathway, etc. It projects to the intermediate nuclei, i.e. globosus, and emboliformis (which in turn send fibers to the red nucleus) and finally reaches the spinal cord via the rubrospinal tract. The pontocerebellum is related to the motor cortex by way of the corticopontocerebellar system. It projects to the dentate nucleus, from there to the ventral lateral nucleus of the thalamus, and finally back to the motor cortex. This area is concerned with coordinating motor activity, particularly of the limbs.

The function of the cerebellum can best be summarized by the word "synergy," thus the deficits resulting from cerebellar disease are related to asynergy. Asynergy is expressed in such conditions as an awkward gait (ataxia), hypotonia, hyporeflexia, dysmetria (missing the mark), jerky and explosive speech, and asthenia. An intention tremor is present when the dentate nucleus or brachium conjunctivum is involved. All signs and symptoms are on the same side as the lesion.

14

Pyramidal System

Classically, the pyramidal system is considered to be the voluntary motor system controlling fine digital movements. The axons of this system arise from pyramidal cells in the fifth layer of the cortex in the precentral gyrus and premotor area (Fig. 22). The fibers descend through the corona radiata, posterior limb of the internal capsule, and occupy the middle three-fifths of the basis pedunculi of the midbrain. From midbrain levels on down through the pons and medulla, fibers leave the main tract and some terminate in motor nuclei of cranial nerves of both sides, constituting the corticobulbar component. Those remaining continue through the basilar portion of the pons. In the medulla the fibers form a compact bundle adjacent to the ventral midline forming the medullary pyramid. In the lower medulla the fibers decussate as fascicles interdigitating with each other. Upon attaining the opposite side they gather in the lateral funiculus of the spinal cord, forming the lateral corticospinal tract, which extends the length of the spinal cord and terminates in the ventral horn. Most of the fibers end in the cervical and lumbosacral enlargements, but a few remain uncrossed and descend as the ventral corticospinal tract in the ventral funiculus. They descend only to lower cervical levels. Most cross to the opposite side and end indirectly in the ventral horn.

There is topographical representation of the body on the

89

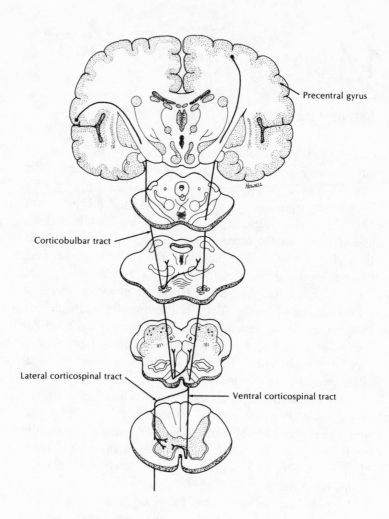

Precentral gyrus

HOWELL

Corticobulbar tract

Lateral corticospinal tract

Ventral corticospinal tract

22. Pyramidal System

precentral gyrus. The head area is located lateroventrally and adjacent to the lateral fissure. The lower extremity is dorsal and medial and the upper extremity intermediate. The area of representation for any group of muscles is directly related to the degree to which they control fine movements, i.e. the finer the movement the greater area of cortex devoted to the muscles responsible for that movement. Most muscles are represented in the contralateral cortex. Some have bilateral representation and others have virtually no representation. In the latter group are those muscles responsible for gross movements (proximal muscles of the trunk and extremities). The muscles with contralateral representation are those of the extremities and lower half of the face. The muscles of mastication, muscles of the tongue, and sternocleidomastoid and trapezius have varying degrees of bilateral representation. The laryngeal and pharyngeal muscles, the muscles in the upper half of the face, and those in the diaphragm are bilaterally represented.

Although some of the fibers of the pyramidal system in higher primates follow the origin, course, and termination outlined above, many others present a different pattern. Fibers descending in the traditional pyramidal pathway arise from a number of areas of the cortex outside the precentral gyrus. The premotor cortex, which is forward to the precentral gyrus, contributes a large number, the primary somesthetic cortex makes a substantial contribution, and other cortical areas have also been implicated.

Most of the fibers of the pyramidal system terminate in areas outside the lower motor neurons. In the spinal cord many fibers end in the intermediate gray and base of the dorsal horn corresponding to laminae IV through VII. As stated in Chapter 12, this neuronal pool is an important integrating center, receiving an input from all motor areas. It in turn projects to the ventral horn. In the brain stem, numerous fibers can be traced into the reticular formation, particularly in areas adjacent to the motor nuclei of cranial nerves. The reticular formation is the integrator at this level. A substantial number of fibers from the pyramidal tract terminate in, or adjacent to, sensory relay nuclei such as the nucleus cuneatus, nucleus gracilis, and descending nucleus of the trigeminal nerve. This provides a feedback to these nuclei from the sensorimotor cortex. Thus the cortex may in some way regulate sensory input.

Lesions of the pyramidal tract cause spastic paralysis and the loss of finer movements. The deep reflexes are exaggerated. Interruption of the pathway above the decussation results in contralateral deficits. If the lesion is in the spinal cord the homolateral musculature is affected; but not all muscles are affected equally, due either to poor or bilateral representation in the cortex. In the trunk and extremities following a unilateral lesion in the cord or brain stem the more distal muscles exhibit the greatest degree of paralysis. However, if the lesion is in the brain stem the effects are contralateral. If the lesion is high in the brain stem, the muscles of the diaphragm, larynx, pharynx, esophagus, upper half of the face, and the extraocular muscles are not affected because of bilateral cortical representation. In this case the contralateral lower half of the face is paralyzed, whereas the opposite muscles of mastication, and of the tongue may show various degrees of involvement.

15

Basal Ganglia and Related Nuclei

The basal ganglia are large nuclear masses (Fig. 23) found at the base of the telencephalon medial to the insula and lateral to the diencephalon, and include the caudate nucleus, putamen, and globus pallidus. The putamen and globus pallidus are frequently referred to as the lenticular nucleus, and the putamen and caudate as the corpus striatum. Some investigators include the claustrum and amygdala in the basal ganglia. The claustrum is a thin lamina of gray matter situated between the extreme and external capsules. The functional relationship to the basal ganglia is not known. It may also be a portion of the insular cortex. The amygdaloid nucleus, which belongs to the olfactory and limbic systems, will be discussed in Chapter 18.

The basal ganglia have extensive connections, both direct and indirect, with the cortex, thalamus, substantia nigra, and subthalamic nucleus. Most of the afferent fibers terminate in the caudate nucleus and putamen, but a few may end directly in the globus pallidus. All cortical areas, particularly the orbital gyri, give rise to corticostriatal fibers. Nuclei of the thalamus (parafascicular and centromedian) give rise to thalamostriatal fibers, which penetrate the internal capsule to terminate primarily in the putamen. The putamen and caudate receive a strong projection from the substantia nigra. Nigrostriatal fibers ascend through the ventral thalamus and penetrate the internal capsule and globus pallidus to end in the putamen and caudate. The

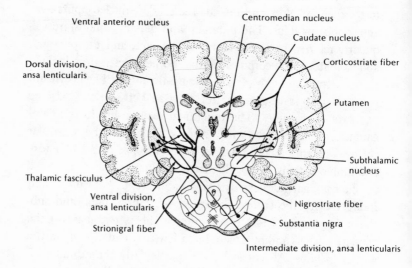

Ventral anterior nucleus

Centromedian nucleus

Caudate nucleus

Dorsal division,
ansa lenticularis

Corticostriate fiber

Putamen

Subthalamic
nucleus

Thalamic fasciculus

Nigrostriate fiber

Ventral division,
ansa lenticularis

Strionigral fiber

Substantia nigra

Intermediate division, ansa lenticularis

23. Basal Ganglia Connections

94

globus pallidus receives a large number of fibers from the sub-thalamic nucleus.

There are numerous interconnections between the nuclei of the basal ganglia. The efferent projections, however, arise mainly from the globus pallidus. Fibers leave the globus pallidus in three streams. One group of fibers penetrates the internal capsule and forms a compact bundle on the dorsal border of the subthalamic nucleus. This is the dorsal division of the ansa lenticularis or lenticular fasciculus. Arising from this tract is the thalamic fasciculus, which turns laterally and dorsal to the lenticular fasciculus to enter the anterior and lateral division of the ventral nucleus of the thalamus. Some fibers leave the thalamic fasciculus to end in the centromedian nucleus. The remaining fibers of the dorsal division of the ansa lenticularis continue caudally, to terminate in the tegmental nuclei.

A second group of fibers from the globus pallidus penetrates the internal capsule and ends in the subthalamic nucleus. This is the intermediate division of the ansa lenticularis or subthalamic fasciculus. The third group is the ventral division of the ansa lenticularis. It is a compact bundle of fibers ventral to the globus pallidus. It loops around the anterior limb of the internal capsule. It then joins the lenticular fasciculus and subsequent distribution is the same as described above. The putamen and caudate nucleus, in addition to having extensive efferent connections with the globus pallidus, project directly to the substantia nigra.

The substantia nigra has further connections with the thalamus and superior colliculus. The latter in turn gives rise to tectospinal fibers. In this way the basal ganglia may influence activity in the tectospinal tract. The ventral anterior and lateral nuclei project to the motor cortex.

Since none of the nuclei usually associated with the basal ganglia send fibers to lower brain stem and spinal levels, with the exception of the nigrotectal-tectospinal system, they must exert their influence on lower motor neurons by way of the cerebral cortex. They therefore modulate motor activity of cortical origin. The basal ganglia are concerned with coarse stereotyped movements. They have their principal influence over the proximal musculature. Even following pyramidal tract destruction the individual may be able to carry out numerous motor acts, such as walking and eating. This system is responsible for the associated movements that support voluntary activities, i.e. swinging the arms while walking, changes of facial expression while talking. It also plays an important role in the maintenance of proper muscle tone and postural adjustments.

Lesions of the basal ganglia or tracts, or other nuclei belonging to this system, cause altered muscle tone, the loss of associated movements, and the appearance of an adventitial movement. The muscle tone is usually increased, resulting in rigidity, which is increased tone in both flexors and extensors. The individual presents a masked expression and except for the adventitial movement there is a paucity of movement. The adventitial movement, which disappears during sleep, may take several forms: there may be rhythmic tremors, slow writhing athetoid movements, or fast jerky choreiform movements.

16

The Reticular Formation

The reticular formation is a diffuse system of nuclei and tracts occupying the central core of the neuraxis from the thalamus to the spinal cord. Phylogenetically, it is the oldest part of the chordate central nervous system. In lower forms it acts as the sole integrator of sensorimotor activity. As the brain increases in complexity, long ascending and descending tracts and associated nuclei appear to develop from the reticular core and assume a peripheral position in the brain stem and spinal cord. In lower forms, most of the ascending tracts terminate in the reticular formation. They attain the thalamus directly only in mammals, but there still remain rich connections of these systems with the reticular formation. Furthermore, a direct corticospinal system can be recognized only in mammals, but even in this group it is poorly developed except in primates. This system also maintains strong corticoreticular connections in mammals, and it is thus apparent that the reticular formation must serve as an important integrator of central nervous system activity.

The cell bodies of the neurons that make up the reticular formation are segmentally arranged in transverse planes; the dendrites branch profusely adjacent to the cell body, whereas the axon usually bifurcates. The ascending limb may ascend as far as the diencephalon, where it terminates in two general areas, i.e. the hypothalamus and the intralaminar thalamic nuclei. It is possible that a few pass directly to the basal ganglia. The descending fibers end on cells around the motor nuclei of cranial nerves and laminae VI–VIII of the spinal cord, making up the diffuse reticulobulbar and reticulospinal tracts respectively—in which there is generally recognized a ventral and lateral tract descending diffusely in the corresponding funiculi of the spinal cord. Crossed and uncrossed fibers are present in both the ascending and descending systems. Throughout the course of these axons numerous collaterals are given off at all levels. These branch profusely and terminate in relation to other reticular neurons as well as in all other nuclei of the brain stem, thus it appears that pathways through the reticular formation are both direct and diffuse.

All ascending and descending tracts send numerous collaterals into all levels of the reticular formation. These terminate in relation to the dendrites and cell bodies of the reticular neurons. In addition there are numerous direct connections from the spinal cord and higher centers, i.e. spinoreticular, corticoreticular, tectoreticular, vestibuloreticular, cerebelloreticular, etc. By this means all sensory modalities reach the reticular formation as do influences from neocortex, limbic lobe, basal ganglia, hypothalamus, thalamus, cerebellum, etc.

The central tegmental fasciculus is the most prominent tract of the reticular formation. In the medulla it can be seen around the inferior olivary nucleus. It assumes a central position in the pons and is located between the central gray and red nucleus in the midbrain. The tract contains both ascending and descending fibers. The former arise from the reticular nuclei and terminate in the subthalamic region and intralaminar nuclei. Various nuclei of the midbrain, e.g. red nucleus, give rise to the descending fibers which terminate largely in the inferior olivary nucleus. The fasciculus also contains numerous short fibers.

It is apparent from the discussion above of the morphology of the reticular formation that it is, either directly or indirectly, in two-way communication with every other area of the central nervous system. This anatomical arrangement is ideal for the reticular formation to perform its most important function of integration.

Although a great deal remains to be determined about the functions of the reticular formation, on the basis of stimulation and ablation experiments and clinical findings it appears that the reticular core exerts an influence over the entire nervous system and in turn has its activity regulated by these same structures. In general, this two-way control takes the form of inhibition and facilitation. However, despite the apparent diffuse arrangement of the reticular formation, anatomical and physiological studies have shown that it is not a homogeneous unit. Certain nuclei of the reticular formation seem to be primarily related to specific areas of the central nervous system, e.g. the lateral reticular nucleus in the medulla has strong two-way connections with the cerebellum.

Three nuclear groups closely related to the reticular formation are the raphe nuclei, periaqueductal gray, and locus ceruleus. The raphe nuclei are adjacent to the midline in the pons and medulla. They are rich in serotonin and have widespread connections. They may play a role in modulating behavior. As previously mentioned, one division, the nucleus raphe magnus, may be important in pain transmission. The periaqueductal gray surrounds the cerebral aqueduct in the midbrain. It seems to be related to the reticular formation, hypothalamus, and certain thalamic nuclei. It is thought to be involved in pain and certain behavioral reactions. The locus ceruleus is a small nucleus found in the upper pons near the floor of the fourth ventricle. It is rich in norepinephrine. Although a small nucleus, its axons have numerous collaterals which reach virtually all parts of the central nervous system. Little is known of its function, but obviously it has widespread influence.

Reticular influences on other areas of the nervous system

may conveniently be discussed under the headings "ascending" and "descending." Stimulation of the reticular core induces arousal in the sleeping animal. The electroencephalographic record in such an experiment abruptly changes from the typical sleeping pattern (slow, high amplitude, regular waves) to that of wakefulness (fast, low amplitude, asynchronous waves). This behavioral response recorded by the electroencephalograph indicates an excitatory influence of the reticular formation on the cortex. Stimulation of afferent systems, particularly somatic and auditory, has the same effect. It has been demonstrated that the effect of sensory stimulation is mediated through the reticular formation by way of collaterals from the direct sensory pathways as well as direct fibers from sensory nuclei. These pathways may be sectioned below the thalamus without interfering with the response. Stimulation of certain areas of the reticular core may also induce sleep. Thus the reticular formation has both an excitatory and inhibitory effect on the cortex.

Bilateral lesions of the reticular system induce permanent coma even though the direct sensory pathways remain intact. Temporary blockage of the reticular activating system may be brought about by using various anesthetics. Conversely, excitant drugs, such as epinephrine, have a stimulating effect. Furthermore, there is fragmentary, although conflicting, evidence that tranquilizers may exert some of their influence through the reticular core.

Descending reticular influences are expressed via the neuromuscular system, sensory receptor and conduction systems, and autonomic effectors. Stimulation of the medullary reticular substance inhibits reflex and cortically induced movements, whereas facilitation is observed upon stimulating the pontomesencephalic tegmentum. Normally the activity of these two centers are in perfect balance, allowing for smooth integration of muscular activity. In order to carry out its motor functions the reticular formation must receive signals from a variety of other centers such as vestibular, cerebellar, pallidal, and cortical.

Facilitatory and inhibitory effects on receptors and sensory conduction pathways have been elicited through stimulation of the reticular formation. The influence on receptors is probably mediated through centrifugal fibers to cutaneous receptors, muscle spindles, cochlea, retina, and olfactory bulb. These centrifugal fibers probably have the effect of altering the threshold of the receptors. Reticular stimulation also inhibits or facilitates synaptic transmission at the relay nuclei of the sensory conduction pathways. These phenomena allow the individual to screen the host of stimuli, to accept some and reject others.

It has long been recognized that stimulation or ablation of various areas of the reticular formation also has an effect on respiration, circulation, temperature regulation, metabolism, and gastrointestinal motility. These autonomic "centers" are poorly localized and are no doubt intimately interrelated with the other functions of the reticular formation.

17

Autonomic Nervous System

The autonomic nervous system (general visceral efferent) innervates smooth muscle, cardiac muscle, and glands. Fibers
supplying skeletal muscles (general somatic efferent) arise from
cell bodies within the central nervous system and pass directly
to the motor end plates. In the autonomic nervous system a
neuron within the central nervous system gives rise to a fiber
which ends on a multipolar cell in a peripheral ganglion. The
axon of this neuron passes to smooth and cardiac muscles and
glands and ends as a naked terminal. Two neurons are involved:
the cell bodies of the preganglionic are located within the central nervous system; and the cell bodies of the postganglionic are
in the autonomic ganglia.

The autonomic nervous system has two divisions: the sympathetic and the parasympathetic. In the sympathetic division
the preganglionics arise from the thoracic and upper lumbar
cord (thoracolumbar outflow). The preganglionics of the parasympathetic division take origin from the brain or sacral cord
(craniosacral outflow). Most visceral organs have a dual innervation. The exceptions are the blood vessels, arrector pili muscles,
and sweat glands.

The preganglionic fibers of the sympathetic system arise from
the intermediolateral cell column in the thoracic and upper
lumbar cord. They exit with the ventral root. After passing
through the intervertebral foramen they leave the spinal nerve

in the communicating rami to enter a chain of ganglia located adjacent to the vertebral bodies. This is the sympathetic trunk, which extends from the base of the occiput to the coccyx. Some of the fibers terminate in these ganglia either at the level they enter or at some distant point after ascending or descending in the trunk. Postganglionics arising from the ganglia of the trunk join all spinal nerves by way of the communicating rami. These are distributed to blood vessels, arrector pili muscles, and sweat glands. Other preganglionics course through the sympathetic trunk to form the splanchnic nerves. These nerves penetrate the diaphragm and end in ganglia located at the origins of the unpaired branches of the aorta. These are the prevertebral ganglia and consist of the coeliac, superior mesenteric, and inferior mesenteric. Postganglionics reach the viscera by following the blood vessels. Postganglionic sympathetics to the head arise from the highest ganglion of the sympathetic trunk, the superior cervical sympathetic ganglion. They reach the effectors in the head largely by following blood vessels.

Four cranial nerves contain preganglionic parasympathetics: oculomotor, facial, glossopharyngeal, and vagus. Those in the oculomotor nerve arise from the Edinger-Westphal nucleus in the midbrain, enter the orbit, and terminate in the ciliary ganglion. Postganglionics supply the ciliary muscle and the constrictor of the pupil. Preganglionics of the facial nerve arise from the superior salivatory nucleus of the lower pons and terminate in the pterygopalatine and submandibular ganglia. From the submandibular ganglion, postganglionics supply the submandibular and sublingual glands. The sphenopalatine ganglion gives rise to postganglionics which enter the lacrimal gland. The inferior salivatory nucleus of the upper medulla gives rise to preganglionics which course with the glossopharyngeal nerve. They terminate in the otic ganglion, from which postganglionics supply the parotid gland.

The vagus nerve is the most important parasympathetic nerve.

103

Its preganglionics arise from the dorsal motor nucleus of the vagus in the medulla and course with the vagus into the thorax and abdomen. The ganglia of this nerve are located adjacent to or in the visceral organ and are very frequently named after that organ, thus there are cardiac, pulmonary, and enteric (in the wall of the gut) ganglia. Postganglionics are short and end on the adjacent cardiac and smooth muscle. The viscera of the pelvis receive parasympathetics from the sacral outflow. Scattered cells within the intermediate gray of sacral segments two through four give rise to preganglionics which exit with the ventral root of the corresponding sacral nerves. They branch from these nerves, forming the nervus erigens, which enters the pelvis. The ganglia are located adjacent to the corresponding organ and the postganglionics supply the smooth muscles of these organs.

The autonomic nervous system has representation in the central nervous system. The most important center for the integration of basic vegetative functions is the hypothalamus (Fig. 24). This is the ventral division of the diencephalon. The hypothalamus contains numerous nuclei, most of which have ill-defined boundaries. Since specific functions are not generally assigned to specific nuclei the hypothalamus is divided into areas: the supraoptic area is the most anterior and is related to the optic chiasma; the tuberal or middle portion is associated with the tuber cinereum; the posterior or mammillary area is related to the mammillary bodies. The hypothalamus may be further divided into medial and lateral areas by the fornix. Related to the hypothalamus both anatomically and functionally is the preoptic area of the telencephalon, which is immediately anterior to the hypothalamus.

The medial forebrain bundle is one of the most important tracts of the hypothalamus. It contains ascending and descending fibers interconnecting the hypothalamus cephalically with olfactory, septal, and limbic areas, and anterior olfactory nucleus

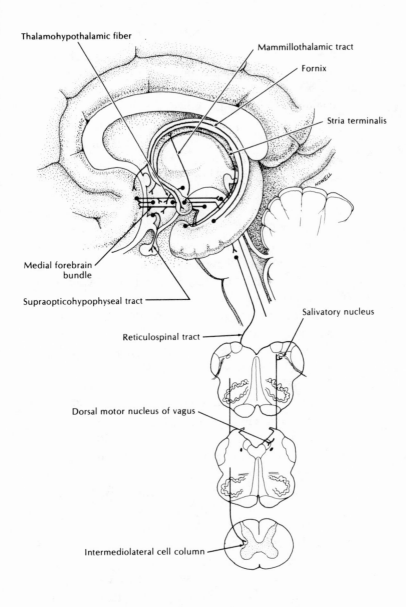

Thalamohypothalamic fiber

Mammillothalamic tract

Fornix

Stria terminalis

Medial forebrain
bundle

Supraopticohypophyseal tract

Salivatory nucleus

Reticulospinal tract

Dorsal motor nucleus of vagus

Intermediolateral cell column

24. Connections of the Hypothalamus

105

and caudally with the tegmentum and reticular formation. The fornix arises from the hippocampus, and parallels the temporal horn and body of the lateral ventricle. Upon reaching the anterior commissure it divides into a precommissural portion, which ends in the preoptic and supraoptic areas, and a post-commissural division, which courses through the hypothalamus to end in the mammillary bodies.

The mammillary peduncle arises from the tegmentum and ascends to terminate in the mammillary bodies and adjacent hypothalamic areas. It also contains some descending fibers. The amygdala projects to the preoptic area and anterior hypothalamus by way of the stria terminalis and ventral amygdalofugal pathway. Finally, the dorsal thalamus, particularly the midline and medial nuclei, sends fibers into the hypothalamus by way of the periventricular system.

A prominent efferent projection of the hypothalamus is the mammillothalamic tract. This tract arises from the mammillary body and terminates in the anterior nucleus of the thalamus, which has extensive connections with the limbic lobe. The supraoptico-hypophyseal tract arises from the supraoptic and paraventricular nuclei, courses through the infundibulum, and ends in the neural lobe. Other ascending fibers pass to the medial nucleus of the thalamus. Still others course in the medial forebrain bundle to end in the septal area and olfactory tubercle. Descending fibers follow two general routes. One group courses diffusely through the reticular formation to reach lower medullary levels. The second descends in the periventricular gray. This includes a discrete bundle, the dorsal longitudinal fasciculus.

As stated previously the hypothalamus is an important integration center of basic vegetative functions which relate to the maintenance of the individual and the species. In order to perform these functions the hypothalamus must receive information from many areas. Afferents from visceral and somatic receptors reach it by way of ascending fiber systems in the reticular formation. Olfaction enters through the medial forebrain bundle. The hypothalamus is intimately related by way of the medial forebrain bundle, fornix, and mammillothalamic tract, to the limbic lobe, which is concerned with emotional tone. Connections with the neocortex are indirect by way of the dorsal thalamus. Finally, certain cells of the hypothalamus are sensitive to the level of some circulating humors.

The hypothalamus utilizes both neural and humoral pathways to reach visceral and somatic effectors and endocrine glands. Descending pathways through the reticular formation and reticulospinal tracts ultimately reach somatic and visceral lower motor neurons. The neurons of the supraoptic and paraventricular nuclei are neurosecretory. They secrete hormones which pass down the supraoptico-hypophyseal tract to the neural lobe of the hypophysis. One of these hormones is the antidiuretic hormone, which regulates the resorption of water by the renal tubules, and it is stored in the neural lobe to be released at the appropriate time. Neurons in the median eminence of the tuberal region secrete certain substances into the hypophyseal portal system which is continuous with the sinuses of the adenohypophysis. The adenohypophysis exerts a marked influence over other endocrine glands via its trophic hormones. By this route the hypothalamus plays an important role in such processes as reproduction and metabolism.

Localization of specific functions within the hypothalamus is difficult. The anterior hypothalamus, however, discharges principally through parasympathetic pathways, whereas stimulation of the posterior regions results in sympathetic responses. The hypothalamus plays a role in temperature regulation: stimulation of the anterior portion produces sweating and vasodilation, and causes heat loss. Other areas of the anterior hypothalamus are concerned with heat production. The hypothalamus is also related to the ascending reticular activating system. Lesions dorsolateral to the mammillary bodies result in somnolence.

Parts of the hypothalamus are concerned with food and water intake. Experiments would indicate that the more medial areas contain a satiety center, whereas feeding behavior is related to the lateral portions.

Emotional behavior is a function of a variety of areas of the central nervous system. The limbic lobe is concerned with emotional tone but, as pointed out above, it has rich connections with the hypothalamus. Certain lesions in the hypothalamus produce irritability and rage. The hypothalamus is the integrator of the effectory mechanisms in emotional expression.

Other areas of the central nervous system will when stimulated give rise to autonomic responses. Stimulation of the cortex, particularly the limbic lobe, produces autonomic responses. These are related to emotional expression and are mediated through the hypothalamus. The brain-stem reticular formation contains centers that regulate the automatic activity of the respiratory and circulatory systems. Their rhythmic activity may be altered by external and internal stimuli and higher centers such as the hypothalamus.

Depending upon the location, lesions of the hypothalamus may result in a variety of signs and symptoms. These are a result of hypothalamic dysfunction and may be expressed as obesity, somnolence, diabetes insipidus, personality change, difficulty in maintaining body temperature, genital dystrophy, sexual precocity, etc.

18

Olfactory and Limbic Systems

The olfactory and limbic systems are discussed together since they are closely related structurally and phylogenetically. The olfactory receptors are actually bipolar neurons located in the olfactory membrane in the roof of the nasal cavity (Fig. 25). The peripheral process is short and extends to the surface. Hair-like processes (cilia) project from the ends of the peripheral fibers. The central processes form the olfactory nerves, which pass through the openings in the cribriform plate to enter the cranial cavity. Sustentacular cells are also found in the olfactory membrane. The free surface of these cells contains a large number of microvilli, which are both supportive and secretory in function. Resting on the cribriform plate is the olfactory bulb. Within the bulb are large neurons called mitral cells as well as smaller tufted cells. Fibers of the olfactory nerve synapse with dendrites of mitral and tufted cells, forming a glomerulus. The axons of the mitral and tufted cells pass back to form the olfactory tract. Found within the deeper layers of the bulb are small granule cells. These are devoid of axons but their dendrites form dendrodendritic synapses with mitral and tufted cells. Efferent fibers to the bulb also synapse on the granule cells. They are thought to be involved in inhibitory circuits within the bulb.

The olfactory tract passes back to the anterior perforated substance. In the base of the tract are located scattered cells which constitute the anterior olfactory nucleus. Some fibers of

109

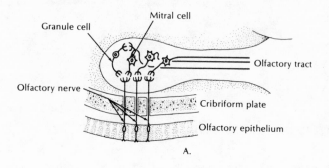

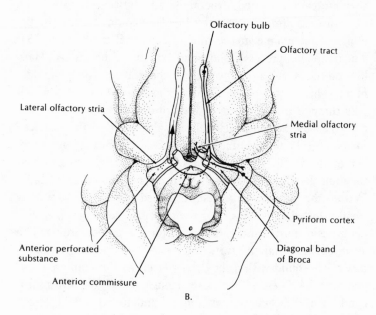

25. Olfactory Bulb and Secondary Olfactory Connections A. detail of olfactory bulb B. underside of brain showing olfactory connections

the olfactory tract terminate here. The anterior olfactory nucleus sends fibers into the olfactory tract. At the rostral border of the anterior perforated substance the olfactory tract divides into medial and lateral olfactory striae. A few fibers of the tract terminate on cells of the anterior perforated substance. This area, which is highly developed in macrosmatic animals, forms the olfactory tubercle.

Associated with each stria is a thin band of gray matter, the medial and lateral olfactory gyri. The lateral olfactory stria courses along the rostral and lateral border of the anterior perforated substance, and at the inferior border of the insula it turns back to enter the temporal lobe. Its fibers terminate in the lateral olfactory gyrus, periamygdaloid area, a portion of the amygdaloid nucleus, and the rostral portion of the parahippocampal gyrus. These constitute the primary olfactory cortex and are known as the pyriform lobe. The lateral olfactory gyrus is frequently referred to as the prepyriform area and the remainder of the pyriform lobe as the entorhinal cortex. This includes the uncus, which is a hook-like rostral end of the parahippocampal gyrus covering the amygdala. Some fibers of the lateral olfactory stria pass back to terminate in the anterior and lateral hypothalamus.

Some fibers of the medial olfactory stria cross in the anterior commissure and terminate in the opposite anterior olfactory nucleus and olfactory bulb, forming another reinforcing circuit. These arise from the anterior olfactory nucleus and not directly from the olfactory bulb. The remaining fibers of the medial olfactory stria enter the medial side of the hemisphere and end in the parolfactory area and subcallosal gyrus (paraterminal gyrus). These constitute what is known as the septal area. The subcallosal gyrus, a thin band of gray matter applied to the underside of the rostrum of the corpus callosum, is separated from the parolfactory area by the posterior parolfactory sulcus.

111

The anterior parolfactory sulcus separates the parolfactory gyrus from the remainder of the medial portion of the hemisphere.

There are three prominent discharge pathways from the olfactory areas cited above to lower centers which may be involved in mediating olfactory reflexes. These same pathways, however, arise in part from regions of the limbic system. The stria terminalis takes origin from the amygdala and follows the medial border of the caudate nucleus to end in the preoptic area and anterior hypothalamus. These areas discharge caudally, as outlined in Chapter 17.

The stria medullaris thalami arises from the septal area, septal nuclei (immediately deep to the septal cortex), and hypothalamus. It arches over the medial nucleus of the thalamus to end in the habenular nucleus of the epithalamus. Some fibers cross in the habenular commissure to reach the opposite habenular nucleus. The habenulopeduncular tract (fasciculus-retroflexus) relays olfactory impulses to the interpeduncular nucleus of the midbrain. This nucleus, located in the roof of the interpeduncular fossa projects to the tegmental nuclei, which contribute fibers to the dorsal longitudinal fasciculus. Olfactory impulses may reach brain-stem nuclei via this tract.

The medial forebrain bundle takes origin from the septal areas and anterior perforated substance and passes back to the pre-optic area, hypothalamus, and midbrain tegmentum; these areas project caudally to various brain-stem nuclei. The medial forebrain bundle also contains ascending fibers arising from the areas cited above and ending in olfactory and limbic regions.

The limbic lobe consists of a number of gyri on the medial surface of the hemisphere encircling the brain stem (Fig. 26). Included within this system are the gyrus cinguli located above the corpus callosum; the parahippocampal gyrus in the medial portion of the temporal lobe; the hippocampus and dentate gyrus, which bulge into the temporal horn of the lateral ventricle; and the hippocampal rudiments (indusium griseum), which

112

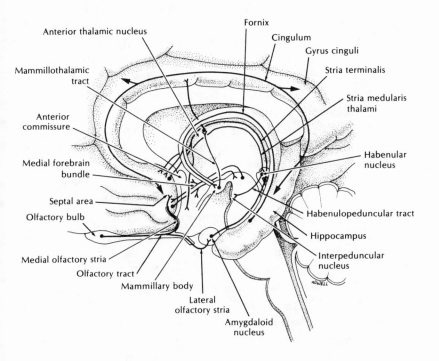

Anterior thalamic nucleus

Fornix

Cingulum

Gyrus cinguli

Mammillothalamic tract

Stria terminalis

Stria medularis thalami

Anterior commissure

Medial forebrain bundle

Habenular nucleus

Septal area

Olfactory bulb

Habenulopeduncular tract

Hippocampus

Medial olfactory stria

Interpeduncular nucleus

Olfactory tract

Mammillary body

Lateral olfactory stria

Amygdaloid nucleus

26. Limbic System

extend over the corpus callosum and septal area. Since a number of cortical areas and subcortical nuclei are functionally related to the limbic lobe, the concept of a limbic system has been introduced. The limbic system includes, in addition to the structures named above, portions of the orbital gyri, insula, septal nuclei, amygdala, preoptic area, hypothalamus, anterior thalamic nucleus, epithalamus, and midbrain tegmentum.

Certain projection pathways relating to the limbic system, namely, stria medullaris thalami, medial forebrain bundle, and stria terminalis, have already been discussed. Other important tracts are the fornix, mammillothalamic tract, anterior commissure, ventral amygdalofugal pathway, and cingulum. The fimbria of the fornix arises from the hippocampus and is attached to the entire length of the hippocampus. At the caudal end of the hippocampus it forms the fornix, which passes into the body of the ventricle; some of the fibers join the opposite fornix. Upon reaching the anterior commissure a smaller precommissural component ends in the septal nuclei, preoptic area, and anterior hypothalamic regions. The larger postcommissural component enters the hypothalamus and terminates in the mammillary body. Some fibers arising from the septal nuclei pass back in the fornix to end in the hippocampus. The mammillothalamic tract passes to the anterior nucleus of the thalamus, which projects to the cortex of the gyrus cinguli.

The anterior commissure is a compact bundle of fibers crossing the midline in the lamina terminalis. Its smaller anterior division is olfactory and interconnects the olfactory bulbs and anterior olfactory nuclei. The posterior division interconnects the prepyriform areas, parahippocampal gyri, and neocortex of the temporal lobe.

The cingulum is an important association bundle of the limbic system. It extends from the septal areas back over corpus callosum, where it forms the white matter of the gyrus cinguli. It turns around the splenium of the corpus callosum to enter

114

the parahippocampal gyrus, and interrelates the septal areas, gyrus cinguli, and parahippocampal gyrus.

The ventral amygdalofugal pathway consists largely of efferent fibers from the amygdaloid nucleus. The dorsal pathway is synonymous with the stria terminalis. These two efferent bundles carry fibers to the hypothalamus, thalamus, neocortex, and brain stem.

All parts of the limbic system are intimately connected with each other, and the system has strong reciprocal connections with the adjacent neocortex. Other afferent projections are from the olfactory areas and the thalamus and hypothalamus. The thalamus and hypothalamus may allow for various somatic and visceral sensory modalities to reach the limbic system.

It is difficult to ascribe any functional localization to specific areas of the limbic system. It appears to regulate emotional tone and influence a wide variety of activities related to emotional tone, such as respiration, cardiac acceleration, chewing and licking motions, various audible sounds such as growling, etc. Stimulation of widely separated points in the limbic system results in these reactions. The common denominator of these responses is that they can be considered as one facet of an emotional expression. The results of lesions support the contention that the limbic system plays a role in regulating emotional tone. Destruction of various areas produce alterations in behavioral mechanisms involved in affective and sexual activities. It appears, therefore, that the limbic lobe is not concerned with the integration of basic homeostatic and adaptive autonomic functions, but rather it modulates emotional tone which is integrated at hypothalamic and brain-stem levels.

Although the integration of effectors in rage and fear is possible without a cortex, true emotional expression is dependent upon a neocortical analyzer. The role of the limbic lobe is to modulate or regulate the emotional tone. Somatoautonomic integration takes place largely at the hypothalamic level. The

115

hypothalamus in turn projects to the appropriate somatic, autonomic, and endocrine effectors.

Clinically the olfactory system is of little importance in man. Anosmia (loss of the sense of smell) may follow frontal fractures that involve the cribriform plate, severing the olfactory nerve. Irritative lesions in the area of the uncus result in olfactory hallucinations known as uncinate fits. Lesions of the limbic system frequently cause behavioral changes. There may be abnormal sexual behavior accompanied by various autonomic changes. Placid behavior follows destruction of the amygdala. The Klüver-Bucy syndrome resulting from bilateral destruction of some of the temporal portion of the limbic lobe is characterized by loss of short-term memory, aberrant sexual behavior, and compulsive feeding behavior.

19

Cerebral Cortex

The neocortex is a thin lamina of gray matter on the surface of the hemisphere, averaging about 2.5 mm in thickness. There are approximately 14,000,000,000 cells within the cortex—of the numerous cell types only the principal ones will be discussed. The most common cells are the pyramidal and stellate (Fig. 27). The pyramidal cells vary from small to giant and have an apical dendrite which extends toward the surface. A basal axon terminates either in the deeper cortical layers or enters the underlying white matter to end in distant cortical areas or subcortical centers. The stellate cell is star-shaped and has numerous short dendrites. The axon, which is also short, does not leave the cortex, and is thus associative in function.

Other neurons in the cortex are the horizontal cells of Cajal, polymorph cells, and cells of Martinotti. The horizontal cells of Cajal are found in the most superficial cortical layer. The dendrites and axon are disposed in a horizontal plane—they are associative in function. The polymorph cells vary in shape from spherical to fusiform and are located in the deepest layers. Their dendrites extend toward the surface. The axon enters the underlying white matter. The cells of Martinotti are found in all layers. Their dendrites are short, and the axon extends toward the surface. They function as association neurons.

On the basis of the distribution of cell types, six cortical layers can be recognized. They are, from superficial to deep:

117

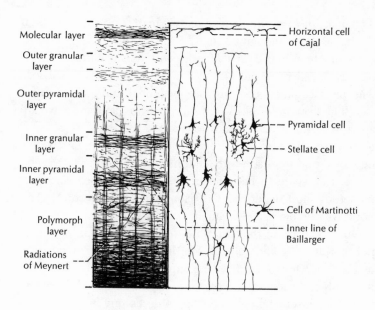

Molecular layer

Outer granular layer

Outer pyramidal layer

Inner granular layer

Inner pyramidal layer

Polymorph layer

Radiations of Meynert

Horizontal cell of Cajal

Pyramidal cell

Stellate cell

Cell of Martinotti

Inner line of Baillarger

After Brodmann (Ranson & Clark)

27. Cerebral Cortex

molecular layer, external granular layer, external pyramidal layer, inner granular layer, inner pyramidal layer, and polymorph layer. The molecular layer contains the horizontal cells of Cajal. The principal constituent, however, is the termination of axons (cells of Martinotti) and dendrites (pyramidal and polymorph cells) of cells in the deeper layers. The principal cell type in the outer granular layer is the small pyramidal cell. Medium-size pyramidal cells dominate the outer pyramidal cell layer. The inner granular layer is composed of stellate cells. Medium, large, and giant pyramidal cells are found in the inner pyramidal layer. Polymorph cells make up the polymorph layer.

In addition to the various cells, certain fiber bands can be recognized in the cortex. The outer line of Baillarger is found within the inner granular layer. It is composed of the terminal ends of afferent fibers, e.g. thalamic radiations. Within the inner pyramidal layer is found the inner line of Baillarger. It is composed of association fibers from other cortical areas. The radiations of Meynert are vertical bundles of fibers formed from axons of pyramidal and polymorph cells entering the white matter.

Although the six cortical layers can be recognized at some stage of development in all areas of the neocortex, they may not be obvious in some regions in the adult. Furthermore there is considerable variation in the development of the various layers. On the basis of pattern of lamination, as many as 250 different areas have been described, and although not conclusively demonstrated in all cases, these variations may reflect functional differences.

In addition to the laminar structure the cortex is also arranged in vertical columns. These columns measure 350–450 μm in diameter. Within these columns the cells and their processes are generally arranged in a radial fashion with a minimal amount of lateral spread. Furthermore the incoming fibers from the thalamus and other areas tend to terminate within the confines of one column. Thus all the cells within one column may respond to the stimulation of one receptor.

The white matter is composed of association, commissural, and projection fibers. The association fibers interconnect cortical areas within one hemisphere. They may be short loops between adjacent gyri or long bundles relating distant points. An example of a short association loop is the stratum calcarinum, which interconnects the cuneus and lingual gyrus. The long association bundles are the cingulum, uncinate fasciculus, superior and inferior longitudinal fasciculi, superior and inferior occipitofrontal fasciculi, and vertical occipital bundle (Fig. 28).

The cingulum was discussed in Chapter 18. The uncinate fasciculus interconnects the cortices of the basal frontal region and temporal pole. The superior longitudinal fasciculus passes back from the frontal lobe above the insula to the parietal, occipital, and temporal regions. The caudal fibers of this bundle run vertically and constitute the vertical occipital bundle. Deep to the superior longitudinal fasciculus is the inferior occipitofrontal fasciculus. This bundle interconnects frontal, temporal, and occipital areas. The inferior longitudinal fasciculus extends from the temporal to the occipital poles. The superior occipitofrontal fasciculus is found between the caudate nucleus and corpus callosum.

The commissural fibers relate the cortices of the two hemispheres and pass through the corpus callosum, which in the midsaggital plane is divided into splenium, body, genu, and rostrum (Fig. 28). Fibers that course through the splenium turn back toward the occipital poles, forming the major forceps. The minor forceps is formed by fibers interconnecting the frontal poles through the genu. The majority of the fibers of the corpus callosum relate association areas and are both symmetrically and asymmetrically connected.

The projection fibers relate the cortex with subcortical centers and are both ascending and descending. They traverse the

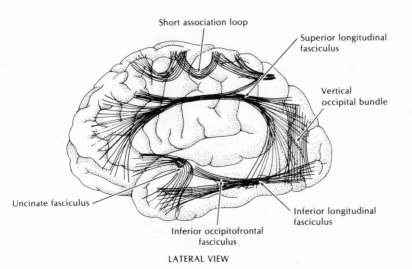

Short association loop

Superior longitudinal
fasciculus

Vertical
occipital bundle

Uncinate fasciculus

Inferior occipitofrontal
fasciculus

Inferior longitudinal
fasciculus

LATERAL VIEW

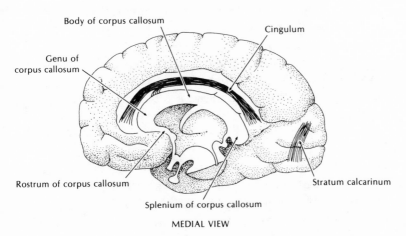

Body of corpus callosum

Cingulum

Genu of
corpus callosum

Rostrum of corpus callosum

Splenium of corpus callosum

Stratum calcarinum

MEDIAL VIEW

28. Association and Commissural Fibers

corona radiata and internal capsule. The internal capsule in a transverse plane has the appearance of a shallow V with the apex directed medially (Fig. 29). The frontothalamic fibers course through the lateral portion of the anterior limb and the frontopontine in the medial portion. The corticobulbar component of the pyramidal system is located in the genu and the corticospinal in the anterior portion of the posterior limb. The somesthetic thalamic radiations ascend through the middle of the posterior limb. Occipitotemporopontine fibers are found in the posterior portion of the posterior limb. The optic radiations assume a retrolenticular position and the auditory radiations, a sublenticular. Other projection fibers, both ascending and descending, connect the cortex with the thalamus, corpus striatum, reticular formation, red nucleus, and substantia nigra, and are diffusely scattered in the internal capsule.

Functionally the cerebral cortex can be divided into primary and association areas. The primary sensory areas receive the thalamic projections of various sensory pathways. The primary somesthetic cortex is located in the postcentral gyrus (Fig. 30). This gyrus extends from the lateral fissure to the medial side of the hemisphere, where, with the medial portion of the precentral gyrus, it forms the paracentral lobule. Separated from the precentral gyrus by the central sulcus, it is the most anterior gyrus of the parietal lobe and receives the somesthetic radiations from the ventral posterior nucleus of the thalamus and projects to association areas. The body is represented somatotopically on the postcentral gyrus. The greater the concentration of receptors in any part of the body the larger the cortical area representing that part. The head area is located adjacent to the lateral fissure, the lower extremity on the medial side of the hemisphere, and the upper extremity intermediate.

The primary visual cortex is located on the medial side of the occipital lobe in the cuneus and lingual gyrus. The optic radiations arising from the lateral geniculate body terminate in the

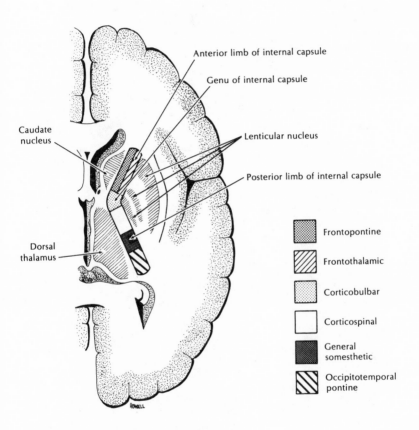

Anterior limb of internal capsule

Genu of internal capsule

Caudate nucleus

Lenticular nucleus

Posterior limb of internal capsule

Dorsal thalamus

Frontopontine

Frontothalamic

Corticobulbar

Corticospinal

General somesthetic

Occipitotemporal pontine

HOWELL

29. Internal Capsule

123

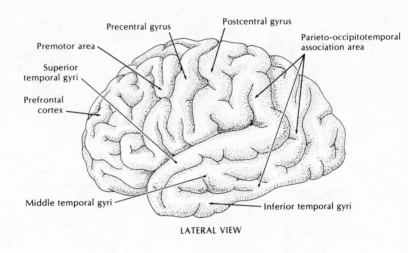

Precentral gyrus Postcentral gyrus
Premotor area Parieto-occipitotemporal association area
Superior temporal gyri
Prefrontal cortex

Middle temporal gyri Inferior temporal gyri

LATERAL VIEW

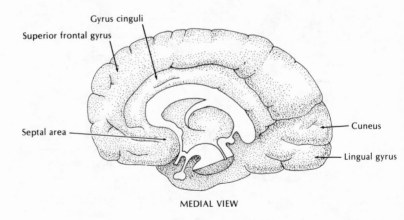

Gyrus cinguli
Superior frontal gyrus

Septal area Cuneus

Lingual gyrus

MEDIAL VIEW

30. Cortical Localization

124

visual cortex. The macular area of the retina is represented in the posterior portion and the more peripheral areas of the retina in the anterior part of the visual cortex.

The primary auditory cortex is located in the transverse temporal gyri on the lower bank of the lateral fissure. The auditory radiations from the medial geniculate body project to this area. Tonotopic localization exists in the auditory cortex. High frequencies are represented posteromedially, and low frequencies, anterolaterally.

The primary gustatory and vestibular areas are not as clearly defined as the other sensory areas. Taste seems to be localized in the insula and adjacent parietal lobe. This area receives a strong projection from the ventral posterior nucleus of the thalamus. Vestibular sensations can be elicited from stimulation of the superior temporal gyrus. These are, however, poorly localized, and other cortical areas have been implicated.

The precentral gyrus constitutes the primary motor cortex. It is closely related functionally and morphologically with the premotor area. There is a somatotopic localization in the precentral gyrus comparable to that found in the postcentral gyrus. It projects primarily into the pyramidal tract. The premotor area, in addition to contributing to the pyramidal tract, has strong connections with the precentral gyrus. It also sends fibers to various subcortical motor nuclei, e.g. basal ganglia, pontine nuclei, reticular formation, etc.

A supplementary motor area as well as secondary sensory areas have been described. These are located adjacent to the corresponding primary area.

The remainder of the cortex is referred to as association cortex. The portion in front of the premotor area is the prefrontal lobe. This area endows the individual with the ability to plan and look to the future; to be persistent in solving a problem; to control his emotions; to deal sociably with others; and to face up to a problem and relate it to past, present, and future experiences.

Patients with lesions of the prefrontal lobes are easily distracted, unable to plan, tactless, extroverted, and without emotional tensions. There may be no loss of basic intelligence, but the ability to abstract is lessened. Prefrontal lobotomies, which involve sectioning the connections of the prefrontal lobes with the rest of the brain, have been performed on psychotic patients and for the relief of intractable pain. Many mentally ill patients have been helped by this procedure, which does not eliminate pain, but rather the patient's anxieties toward pain, and thus he becomes indifferent to it.

The posterior parietal, lateral occipital, and posterior temporal cortices constitute a large association area. It may be referred to as a gnostic center. It is concerned with motor speech and understanding the spoken and written word and the appreciation of symbolism. Portions of the temporal lobe in conjunction with subcortical centers play a role in memory.

Certain lesions in the parietal, occipital, and temporal areas, particularly on the dominant hemisphere may cause apraxia, aphasia, and agnosia. Apraxia is the inability to perform certain complex learned motor acts. However, there is no paralysis or other motor impairment and automatic and associated movements are normal. Aphasia is the loss of ability to use signs and symbols in communication. Expressive aphasia is the inability to express one's thoughts either by speaking or writing. Receptive aphasia is the inability to appreciate the spoken or written word. Agnosia is the inability to recognize and interpret what is felt, seen, or heard.

20

Meninges and Cerebrospinal Fluid

The brain and spinal cord are separated from the bony walls of the cranial cavity and vertebral canal by three fibrous membranes, collectively called the meninges. They are named, from without inward, the dura mater, arachnoid mater, and pia mater (Figs. 31 and 32). The dura mater or pachymenix is a strong non-elastic membrane usually described as consisting of two layers: external endosteal and internal meningeal. The outer endosteal layer is tightly adherent to the inner surface of the cranial vault and is continuous with the pericranium at the foramen magnum and cranial nerve foramina. The meningeal layer follows the inner contours of the skull and is tightly joined to the endosteal layer except at the sites of the venous sinuses and where it is reflected inward to form partitions between various portions of the brain. These fibrous partitions are called the falx cerebri, tentorium cerebelli, falx cerebelli, and diaphragma sellae (Fig. 32B). The sickle-shaped falx cerebri is attached to the entire length of the calvaria at its midline and projects into the longitudinal fissure as a concave fibrous septum separating the cerebral hemispheres. Rostrally, the falx cerebri is securely attached to the crista galli of the ethmoid bone. The superior attached border continues backward to terminate on the internal occipital protuberance. Located within the superior attached border of the falx cerebri is the endothelial-lined superior sagittal sinus. The concave or free border is closely associated with the

127

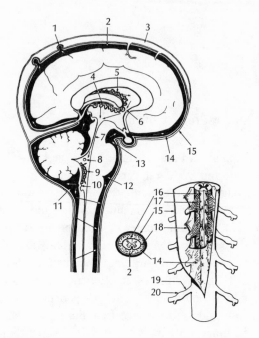

1	arachnoid villi
2	subarachnoid space
3	superior sagittal sinus
4	choroid plexus of the third ventricle
5	choroid plexus of the lateral ventricle
6	interventricular foramen
7	cerebral aqueduct
8	lateral foramen (of Luschka)
9	choroid plexus of the fourth ventricle
10	median foramen (of Magendie)
11	cisterna magna
12	pontine cistern
13	interpeduncular cistern
14	arachnoid mater
15	dura mater
16	pia mater
17	dorsal root
18	dentate ligament
19	spinal nerve
20	dorsal root ganglion

31. Meninges and Cerebrospinal Fluid

From *Pathology of the Nervous System*, Vol. I, edited by J. Minckler et al. Copyright © 1967 by McGraw-Hill, Inc. Used by permission of McGraw-Hill Book Company.

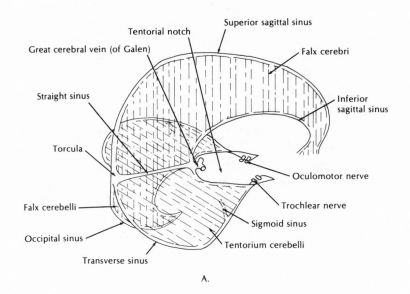

Tentorial notch

Superior sagittal sinus

Great cerebral vein (of Galen)

Falx cerebri

Straight sinus

Inferior
sagittal sinus

Torcula

Oculomotor nerve

Trochlear nerve

Falx cerebelli

Sigmoid sinus

Occipital sinus

Tentorium cerebelli

Transverse sinus

A.

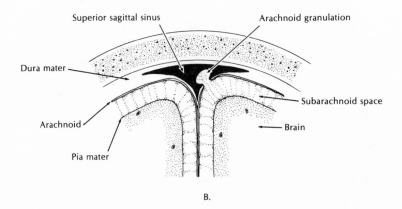

Superior sagittal sinus

Arachnoid granulation

Dura mater

Subarachnoid space

Arachnoid

Brain

Pia mater

B.

32. Meninges and Dural Sinusus A. reflections of the dura mater and associated sinuses B. frontal section through superior sagittal sinus

superior surface of the corpus callosum. Directly behind the splenium of the corpus callosum it fuses along the superior midline surface of the horizontally placed tentorium cerebelli. The free concave edge of the falx cerebri contains the inferior sagittal sinus. This sinus continues backward to join the straight sinus located along the midline where the falx cerebri and tentorium cerebelli are joined. The tentorium cerebelli forms a roof over the posterior cranial fossa and thereby separates the superior surface of the cerebellum from the occipital lobes of the cerebral hemispheres. The outer circumferential border of the tentorium cerebelli is attached to the occipital bone along a groove which contains the transverse or lateral venous sinus and along the lips of a groove located on the superior aspect of the petrous portion of the temporal bone. This latter groove affords passage for the superior petrosal sinus. The outer border then continues forward to terminate on the paired posterior and anterior clinoid processes of the sphenoid bone. An opening is present along the midline of the tentorium cerebelli at this level. It is deeply concave and, together with the dorsum sellae, forms the tentorial notch, which is occupied by the midbrain. The diaphragma sellae is a quadrangular portion of the meningeal dura which roofs over the hypophyseal fossa except for a small central aperture that allows the passage of the stalk of the pituitary gland. Its outer attached border contains the circular venous sinus. The falx cerebelli is a small triangular reflection of the meningeal layer of dura mater situated directly below the internal occipital protuberance. The outer border is anchored along the midline of the occipital bone and contains the occipital sinus. The free border of the falx cerebelli may project inwardly a short distance between the cerebellar hemispheres.

The inner meningeal layer of the dura mater continues as a tubular extension through the foramen magnum. Although the spinal cord ends at approximately the upper part of the second lumbar vertebra, the dural tube continues caudally to terminate in a cul-de-sac at the second sacral vertebra. It loosely invests the spinal cord; and unlike the cranial dura, a space is found between the meningeal layer and the outer periosteal layer. This space is called the extradural space and is filled with a meshwork of areolar tissue and fat. It also contains blood vessels associated with the walls and contents of the vertebral canal.

The arachnoid and pia mater are two thin membranes united by trabeculae of connective tissue. The space between these two layers is called the subarachnoid space and is filled with cerebro-spinal fluid (CSF). The term "leptomeninges" is sometimes applied to the combination of the arachnoid mater and pia mater. The arachnoid mater, as the name implies, is a delicate web-like membrane lying deep to the meningeal layer of dura mater in the craniovertebral cavities, but separated from this last layer by a potential subdural space. Since the arachnoid membrane does not dip down into the various depressions on the surface of the brain, the subarachnoid space is variable in size. These spaces are quite large in some areas and are termed "cisterns," e.g. pontine, interpeduncular, and cisterna magna. The spinal arachnoid space is quite uniform except where it envelops the lower end of the spinal cord and cauda equina to form the lumbar cistern. The pia mater, on the other hand, closely invests the surface of the brain and spinal cord. This close attachment is made possible by the fusion of the pia mater with a marginal layer of glia cells and is referred to as the pia-glial membrane. The cerebral blood vessels must cross the subarachnoid space in order to enter the brain and spinal cord. The vessels are thus surrounded for some distance by a perivascular sheath composed of the leptomeninges. The inner layer of this perivascular sheath is formed by a condensation of the arachnoid and is firmly attached to the adventitia of the vessel, while the outer layer is a continuation of the pia-glial membrane. The two layers of this

131

sheath are separated from each other by a cerebrospinal fluid-filled cleft called the perivascular (Virchow-Robin) space. This space is present around all larger surface vessels. Electron microscopic studies have shown that, as the vessels penetrate more deeply, the two layers fuse to form a cul-de-sac at the level of the terminal arterioles and small venules. These spaces have not been identified by electron microscopy around either the brain capillaries or neurons.

The pial covering of the spinal cord presents a thickened narrow band along the crest of the anterior fissure referred to as the linea splendens. Along the lateral surface of the spinal cord the pia extends outwardly as a lateral longitudinal ridge. This is termed the "ligmentum denticulatum." It is attached firmly to the inner surface of the dura mater and arachnoid by a series of pointed processes which project out between the dorsal and ventral roots of the spinal nerves. Normally, there are 21 pairs of these projections, extending from the foramen magnum to the termination of the spinal cord. At the tip of the spinal cord, the pia continues inferiorly as a slender strand of fibrous tissue, the filum terminale, which pierces the lower end of the arachnoid and dural tube to fuse with the periosteum of the dorsal portion of the coccyx. The ligmenta denticulata and the filum terminale subserve a supporting function for the spinal cord.

As the spinal and cranial nerves pass from the cord and brain through their respective foramina, they are invested for a short distance by the meninges. Along the exiting spinal nerves the dura mater ensheathes both the dorsal and ventral roots to fuse with the epineurium adjacent to the distal portion of the dorsal root ganglia. The arachnoid also forms a separate sheath for both roots and terminates near the proximal portion of the dorsal root ganglia, while the pia contributes the innermost layer around each nerve root and is prolonged into the intervertebral foramen and then blends with the epineurium. The same general arrangement persists for most of the cranial nerves. The optic nerve is an exception since it is an extension of the central nervous system and is, therefore, completely surrounded by the three meningeal layers and associated subarachnoid space.

The cerebrospinal fluid is a clear and colorless fluid having properties similar to the aqueous humour of the eye. Normally, the CSF contains small amounts of protein and glucose, a few lymphocytes, and rather high concentrations of potassium and sodium chloride, which are probably important in keeping CSF in osmotic equilibrium with the blood. The specific gravity of the brain is close to that of water, since it weighs 1500 g in air and approximately 50 g in CSF. The major purpose usually assigned to the CSF is to cushion the brain within the cranial cavity. The fluid also has an important functional role with reference to the nutrition of the central nervous system and the removal of products of metabolism. It also has been shown to contain biologically active substances such as neurohormones and various transmitters. The sites of production and the physiological significance of these substances are the subject of many clinical and experimental studies. The bulk of CSF is produced by the secretory activity of specialized structures called the choroid plexuses, which are located in the lateral, third and fourth ventricles of the brain. Since the CSF is more or less continually formed in the lateral ventricles, it must circulate through the interventricular foramina and, with that produced in the third ventricle, pass through the cerebral aqueduct of the midbrain to the fourth ventricle. Additional fluid is added here from the choroid plexuses of the fourth ventricle and this, coupled with other fluid, escapes by way of one median and two lateral foramina located in the roof of the fourth ventricle into the subarachnoid space. In addition to the fluid produced by the choroid plexuses, there is evidence to suggest an extrachoroidal source of fluid which is similar in composition to that of the choroidal CSF. It is presumed that the extrachoroidal fluid has its site of formation in the pia-glial junctions and thus enters both the

133

ventricles and the subarachnoid space. The circulation of the CSF is sluggish and its movement is regulated, at least in part, through the ventricular-subarachnoid system by hydrostatic gradients. Exactly how the CSF returns to the venous circulation is debatable. It is generally assumed that a major portion leaves the cerebrospinal fluid system by way of channels located in the arachnoid granulations. These structures are finger-like projections of arachnoid membrane that extend into the lumen of the superior sagittal sinus (Fig. 32B). Especially large arachnoid granulations (Pacchionian bodies) are also found in lateral extensions of the superior sagittal sinus and may be especially large in older individuals. A significant amount of fluid may also reach the venous system in still other ways, such as along the cerebrospinal nerve roots or possibly directly from the subarachnoid space.

The spinal cord ends approximately at the second lumbar vertebra, while the subarachnoid space surrounding the lower spinal nerves (cauda equina) continues to the level of the second sacral vertebra. A needle introduced into the subarachnoid space (lumbar cistern) below the tip of the spinal cord affords an opportunity to measure the cerebral spinal fluid pressure or to inject substances into the CSF system, i.e. anesthetics or contrast media. Small amounts of fluid can be removed for serological and chemical tests.

Estimates of the total volume of CSF in the adult vary between 100 and 160 ml and the total volume is thought to be renewed every six to eight hours. Under certain pathological conditions an excessive accumulation of fluid within the CSF system sometimes occurs. This is called hydrocephalus and may arise as a consequence of one or a combination of the following disturbances: by overproduction of CSF; by an obstruction at some point in the cerebrospinal fluid pathway; or from impairment of the absorption pathways.

21

Cerebral Circulation

The brain receives its blood supply from two paired arteries: the internal carotids and vertebrals (Figs. 33 and 34). The vertebral arteries pierce the spinal dura and arachnoid between the base of the skull and atlas to enter the posterior cranial fossa through the foramen magnum. At this level they move toward the ventral surface of the brain stem and join to form a single vessel, the basilar artery. This vessel continues rostrally to terminate by dividing into two posterior cerebral arteries at the superior border of the pons. Each posterior cerebral artery is connected, by a posterior communicating artery, to the corresponding internal carotid artery. On reaching the base of the skull, the internal carotid arteries enter the carotid canals, situated in the petrous portion of the temporal bone, and continue upward through the cavernous sinus to emerge within the middle cranial fossa lateral to the optic chiasma. Anatomically the vertebral and internal carotid arteries are two separate systems which are connected by varying degrees through an anterior and two posterior communicating arteries. Thus, these various branches at the base of the brain form an arterial circle, the circle of Willis. There are, however, a number of anatomical variations in this vascular circle and some of the communicating branches may be absent or vary considerably in size. Normally the communications between these two arterial systems are extensive enough so

135

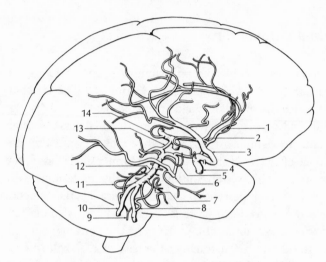

1	anterior cerebral artery	8	posterior inferior cerebellar artery
2	anterior communicating artery	9	anterior spinal artery
3	middle cerebral artery	10	vertebral artery
4	internal carotid artery	11	anterior inferior cerebellar artery
5	superior cerebellar artery	12	basilar artery
6	posterior cerebral artery	13	posterior communicating artery
7	internal auditory artery	14	anterior choroidal artery

33. Arterial Supply of the Brain

From *Pathology of the Nervous System*, Vol. I, edited by J. Minckler et al. Copyright © 1967 by McGraw-Hill, Inc. Used by permission of McGraw-Hill Book Company.

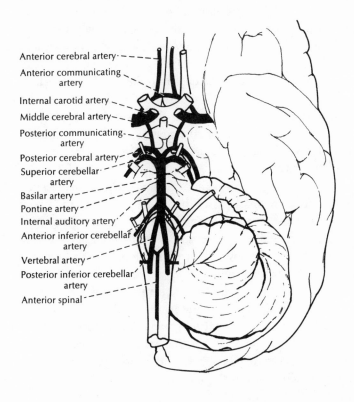

Anterior cerebral artery

Anterior communicating artery

Internal carotid artery

Middle cerebral artery

Posterior communicating artery

Posterior cerebral artery

Superior cerebellar artery

Basilar artery

Pontine artery

Internal auditory artery

Anterior inferior cerebellar artery

Vertebral artery

Posterior inferior cerebellar artery

Anterior spinal

34. Arterial Supply of the Brain (ventral view)

that blood flow to the brain is not impaired if one of the major vessels is interrupted.

The posterior inferior cerebellar arteries arise from the vertebral arteries shortly after they enter the cranial cavity and pass dorsally, winding around the medulla, to the inferior surface of the cerebellum. They supply the dorsal lateral portion of the medulla as well as the inferior surface of the cerebellum. In its course along the ventral surface of the pons, the basilar artery gives rise to a medial and lateral group of pontine arteries. The medial group penetrates the midline of the pons to supply the pyramidal tract, medial lemniscus, medial longitudinal fasciculus, and the third, fourth, and sixth cranial nerve nuclei. The lateral group supplies the middle cerebellar peduncle, facial nucleus, and the trigeminal nucleus. The anterior inferior cerebellar artery arises from the basilar artery in the lower half of the pons. It courses dorsally, supplying the middle cerebellar peduncle, some of the vestibular nuclei, and the anterior and inferior portions of the cerebellum. Just before the basilar artery bifurcates into the posterior cerebrals, the superior cerebellar arteries are given off. As each vessel passes the lateral surface of the upper pons it supplies the spinal lemniscus and then enters the cerebellum, supplying its superior surface and most of the deep cerebellar nuclei. The posterior cerebral arteries are the terminal branches of the basilar artery. They pass backward and over the cerebral peduncle to reach the inferior surface of the cerebral hemispheres where they distribute mainly to the medial and inferior surface of the occipital lobe and inferior surface of the temporal lobe. The posterior cerebral arteries also give rise to a number of penetrating branches that supply portions of the thalamus, cerebral peduncle, internal capsule and the choroid plexuses of the lateral and third ventricles. The posterior communicating arteries, which extend from the posterior cerebrals to the internal carotid, supply portions of the optic chiasma, subthalamic region, basis pedunculi, internal capsule, and thalamus.

138

The basilar artery, in addition to its branches to the brain, also gives rise to the slender internal auditory artery which accompanies the eighth cranial nerve to supply the inner ear.

The ophthalmic artery arises from the internal carotid immediately after it enters the cranial cavity. It passes through the optic foramen and runs forward and laterally below the optic nerve to enter the orbit. The anterior choroidal artery is a small branch which arises close to the junction of the posterior communicating and internal carotid artery. This vessel passes backward along the optic tract and supplies the posterior portion of the choroid plexus of the lateral ventricle and portions of the optic tract and radiations, amygdaloid nucleus, caudate nucleus, basis pedunculi, lenticular nucleus, and anterior commissure.

After giving off the branches named above, each internal carotid artery divides into two principal terminal vessels, the anterior cerebral and middle cerebral. The paired anterior cerebral arteries pass forward and medially above the optic chiasma and at this level are interconnected by the anterior communicating artery. Each vessel then continues forward and dorsally around the genu of the corpus callosum and then posteriorly above the body of the corpus callosum, terminating in the region of the parieto-occipital fissure, where it may anastomose with the terminal branches of the posterior cerebral artery. The main trunk of each anterior cerebral artery supplies branches to the anterior medial and the superior lateral aspects of the cerebral hemispheres. Numerous small perforating branches leave the anterior cerebral arteries near their origins and pass through the anterior perforated substance to supply the cephalic portions of the internal capsule and corpus striatum. A basal branch, the medial striate artery (recurrent artery of Heubner), supplies small areas of the basal ganglia and internal capsule.

The remaining, and larger, of the two terminal branches of the internal carotid artery is the middle cerebral artery. This vessel passes into the lateral fissure and distributes numerous branches along its course to its corresponding hemisphere. In its course through the lateral fissure, the middle cerebral artery supplies the cortex of the insula as well as the opercular and lateral surfaces of the frontal, parietal, and temporal lobes (including the transverse temporal gyri). Small central branches arise near the base of this vessel, the medial and lateral striate arteries, which supply portions of the globus pallidus, internal capsule, and caudate nucleus. One of the lateral striate branches, which supplies a large area of the basal ganglia and internal capsule, is often prone to rupture in older people. For this reason it is referred to as the artery of cerebral hemorrhage.

In general, it may be stated that anastomoses do not occur between the cortical and penetrating branches of the cerebral arteries. There may or may not be anastomoses between neighboring cortical vessels. In any case, they are seldom sufficient to maintain nutrition of the area if one of the vessels is occluded. The central branches of the cortical vessels may occasionally show anastomoses, but these too are rarely adequate. The brain accounts for only 3 per cent of the body weight and in the resting state receives one-sixth of the cardiac output and consumes approximately 20 per cent of the body oxygen.

The spinal cord is supplied by the two dorsal spinal arteries and the single ventral spinal artery. The latter arises as two trunks from the vertebral arteries, which anastomose ventrally and descend in the ventral median fissure of the spinal cord. Throughout its extent its flow is augmented by communicating vessels passing through the intervertebral foramina that arise from the systemic circulation. The anterior spinal arteries supply approximately the ventral two-thirds of the spinal cord. The posterior spinal arteries arise from either the vertebral arteries or the posterior inferior cerebellar arteries. They are small, frequently disconnected arteries that descend adjacent to the point of entrance of the dorsal spinal roots. They also communicate with the systemic circulation through each of the intervertebral foramina. Collectively they supply the dorsal one-third of the spinal cord.

The venous outflow of the brain can be arbitrarily divided into a superficial and deep system of veins. The superficial veins essentially drain the cortical and adjacent subcortical areas of the brain, while the more deeply placed veins drain the basal ganglia, thalamus, and hypothalamus. The veins associated with the cerebral cortex are divided into an inferior and into a superior system. The superior portion is divided into frontal, precentral, postcentral, and occipital groups, which drain into the superior sagittal sinus (Figs. 32A and 35). The ventrolateral surface of the cerebral cortex and inferior surface of the frontal, temporal, and occipital lobes are drained by the inferior cerebral veins. These empty into various sinuses: the superior and inferior petrosal, cavernous, transverse, and sphenoparietal sinuses, and also the vena cerebri magna.

The deep white matter of the cerebral hemispheres and portions of the basal ganglia, choroid plexuses, dorsal thalamus, and hypothalamus are drained by the paired internal cerebral veins. These vessels continue posteriorly and unite at the level of the pineal body to form the vena cerebri magna. This vascular complex also receives collaterals from the basal vein which drains portions of the insular region and corpus striatum. Other diencephalic structures are drained by penetrating veins that pass through the anterior and posterior perforated substance to empty into the cavernous sinus or basilar plexus. As in the case of other organs of the body, the venous drainage of the brain is subject to considerable variation. This, coupled with extensive anastomotic connections between the deep and superficial groups of veins, affords numerous collateral pathways for venous discharge. Furthermore, the intracerebral venous system is also connected with veins of the face and scalp. These interconnecting vessels are called emissary veins and are of some clinical importance in that they do not contain valves and thus may serve as

141

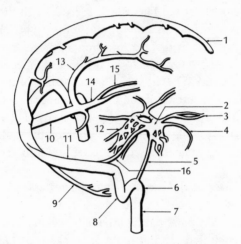

1	superior sagittal sinus	9	occipital sinus
2	cavernous sinus	10	straight sinus
3	ophthalmic veins	11	transverse sinus
4	sphenoparietal sinus	12	basilar venous plexus
5	inferior petrosal sinus	13	inferior sagittal sinus
6	jugular bulb	14	great cerebral vein
7	internal jugular vein	15	internal cerebral vein
8	sigmoid sinus	16	superior petrosal sinus

35. Venous Drainage of the Brain

routes for infectious agents to pass from outside the cranium into the intracranial venous sinuses.

The superior sagittal sinus arises from an emissary vein which communicates with veins of the nasal cavity through the foramen caecum. The superior sagittal sinus passes backwards within the dura of the attached margin of the falx cerebri to the confluens of the sinuses. This latter structure is a dilatation found at the junction of the falx cerebri and tentorium cerebelli. It communicates with the superior sagittal sinus, the straight sinus, the paired transverse sinuses, and the occipital sinus. The inferior sagittal sinus courses posteriorly in the free margin of the falx cerebri and in its course drains the corpus callosum and adjacent medial cortical areas. It terminates by joining with the vena cerebri magna and together they form the straight sinus. This sinus in turn continues posteriorly in the midline of the tentorium cerebelli to empty into the confluens of the sinuses. The superior portion of the cerebellum drains into the straight sinus.

A small marginal sinus surrounds the border of the foramen magnum and is drained by the occipital sinus, which in turn communicates with the internal vertebral venous plexus and thereby connects the vertebral venous plexus with the intracranial sinuses. The transverse sinuses subserve the function of draining the confluens of the sinuses. They pass laterally to the point where the petrous portion meets the squamous portion of the temporal bone. Here they turn ventrally, passing in a groove at the base of the posterior slope of the petrous portion and thus forming the sigmoid sinuses. They terminate by emptying into the jugular bulb which is found within the jugular foramen. Leading from this bulb is the internal jugular vein.

The cavernous sinuses are located one on either side of the sella turcica and are interconnected by the anterior and posterior intercavernous sinuses situated in the anterior and posterior margins of the diaphragma sellae. In addition, the cavernous sinuses receive the venous drainage from the superior (circular sinus)

143

ophthalmic veins and sphenoparietal sinuses. Some of the penetrating veins arising from the base of the brain and a few of the veins draining the cerebral cortex, also empty into the cavernous sinuses. The cavernous sinuses drain by way of the superior and inferior petrosal sinuses. Each superior petrosal sinus extends back over the crest of the petrous portion of the temporal bone to empty into the sigmoid sinus at its junction with the transverse sinus. The inferior petrosal sinus passes back in a groove formed by the petro-occipital suture to empty into the jugular bulb. It receives the major venous drainage from the inferior portion of the cerebellum. The unpaired basilar plexus, located on the clivus of the skull, has connections with the cavernous sinus and also communicates with the vertebral venous system, a system of veins which extends throughout the length of the spinal canal in the epidural space. These veins drain the contents of the spinal canal and communicate at every intervertebral foramen with the systemic circulation. The spinal cord is drained directly by a single anterior spinal vein which accompanies the corresponding artery, and by small discontinuous posterior spinal veins which accompany the comparable arteries. These in turn drain into the vertebral venous system. The vertebral venous system is devoid of valves and has a very low hydrostatic pressure. These points, associated with the fact that the vertebral venous system communicates at all intervertebral levels with the systemic circulation, make this system an ideal pathway for the spread of aberrant metastases and infections.

The central nervous system is unique in that various substances in the blood are prevented from penetrating the environs of the brain and spinal cord. This is probably accomplished, at least in part, by various types of junctions located between the cells that separate the brain pericellular fluid channels from the blood. This barrier mechanism, of which the capillary endothelium, basement membrane, and pericapillary glia sheaths have been implicated (Fig. 36), are very important in establishing a

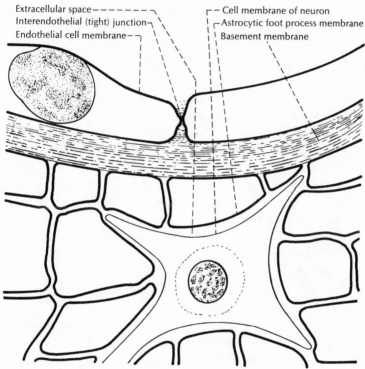

CAPILLARY LUMEN

Extracellular space
Interendothelial (tight) junction
Endothelial cell membrane

Cell membrane of neuron
Astrocytic foot process membrane
Basement membrane

36. Possible Anatomical Sites of the Blood–Brain Barrier

concentration gradient of large molecules between blood and brain. This barrier phenomenon serves in part to protect the neurons from possible noxious substances and it is generally agreed that there is a barrier between blood and brain tissue, i.e. blood–brain barrier; and between the blood and cerebrospinal fluid, i.e. blood–cerebrospinal fluid barrier. There are however areas of the brain that are devoid of a barrier mechanism, e.g. the area postrema, pineal body, and the subcommissural organ.

The existence of interstitial spaces surrounding the neurons and neuroglia is well documented. The spaces are filled with a thin layer of fluid on the order of 150–200 Å in thickness. These fluid-filled spaces communicate via extracellular channels with the ventricular and subarachnoid compartments. The cerebral interstitial fluid, CSF, and the membranes making up the barrier mechanism play an important role in the regulation of the cellular environment of the central nervous system. This is of practical significance since it may act as a hindrance to the effective action of drugs on the central nervous system. Recent evidence suggests that osmotic changes in the blood may shrink or deform the cells at the level of the barrier complex which may alter the effectiveness of the barrier. In addition, tensile stresses such as hypertension or vasodilation may also cause functional alterations in the barrier. High-resolution electron microscopic studies have shown that the intercellular space between the endothelial cells of the cerebral capillaries forms an almost continuous impermeable junction between successive cells. This would imply that small molecules such as glucose would have difficulty passing the blood–brain barrier. However, glucose passes easily from blood to brain, indicating a different mechanism of molecular transport. Therefore all transport across the blood–brain barrier does not necessarily occur at the capillary endothelium and indeed other processes such as carrier mediation may play a role in controlling the composition of cerebral interstitial fluid.

146

22

Clinical Applications

LESIONS OF THE SPINAL CORD

When the dorsal funiculi are involved bilaterally (tabes dorsalis) there is a loss of position sense below the level of the lesion (Fig. 37A). The patient is ataxic (unstable gait) and must watch his lower extremities while walking. There is also a loss of deep tendon reflexes, tactile discrimination, and vibratory sense. The above deficits result from the interruption of the primary nueron in the pathway for proprioception, vibratory sense, and tactile discrimination as discussed in Chapter 5.

Interruption of the decussating pain and temperature fibers in the cord (syringomyelia) results in a bilateral segmental loss of these modalities (Fig. 37B). Since the spinothalamic tracts in the lateral funiculi are spared, there is no loss of pain and temperature above or below the lesion. However, the primary fiber may ascend and descend for as many as two segments before terminating. Therefore the deficit will not extend over as many segments as the lesion (see Chapter 4 for a detailed description of the pain pathways). The degenerative process is progressive and will eventually involve other structures such as the ventral horn cells, pyramidal tracts, etc.

Hemisection of the spinal cord (Brown-Sequard syndrome) may result from stab wounds, lateral compression of the cord by a tumor, etc. (Fig. 37C). The lateral spinothalamic tract is

147

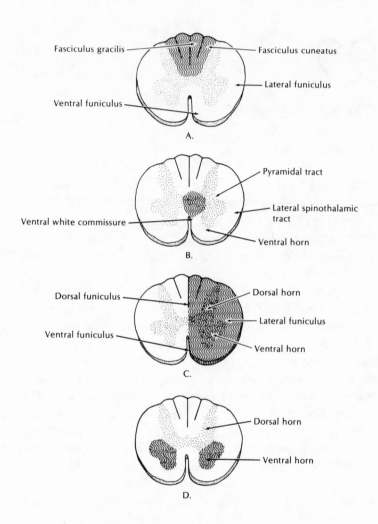

Fasciculus gracilis — Fasciculus cuneatus

Lateral funiculus

Ventral funiculus —

A.

Pyramidal tract

Ventral white commissure — Lateral spinothalamic tract

Ventral horn

B.

Dorsal funiculus — Dorsal horn

Lateral funiculus

Ventral funiculus — Ventral horn

C.

Dorsal horn

Ventral horn

D.

37. Lesions of the Spinal Cord

148

interrupted resulting in contralateral loss of pain and temperature senses beginning about two segments below the level of the lesion. There is homolateral spastic paralysis with increased deep tendon reflexes and a positive Babinski due to the involvement of the pyramidal tract. Homolateral loss of proprioception and vibratory sense below the level of the lesion follows interruption of the dorsal funiculus. If the lesion extends over several segments, flaccid paralysis of the muscles supplied by the ventral horn cells in those segments may occur.

When the ventral horn cells are involved, as in poliomyelitis (Fig. 37D), the skeletal muscles innervated by the diseased neurons are cut off from all neuronal influence. There is a flaccid paralysis, absence of all reflexes, and progressive muscular atrophy. This is an example of a lower motor neuron lesion and is in contrast to one involving an upper motor neuron (pyramidal tract) where there is spastic paralysis and exaggerated deep tendon reflexes.

LESIONS OF THE BRAIN STEM

The deficits resulting from occlusion of the posterior inferior cerebellar artery (Wallenberg's syndrome) are numerous. This artery supplies the dorsolateral aspects of the medulla as well as a portion of the cerebellum (Fig. 38A). There is an inability to perceive pain and temperature change in the opposite arm, trunk and leg due to interruption of the crossed spinothalamic tract. The uncrossed fibers of the descending root of the trigeminal nerve are also involved, resulting in the inability to perceive pain and temperature change in the face on the same side as the lesion. Vertigo, nausea and vomiting, and nystagmus are a consequence of vestibular nuclear involvement. The exiting fibers of cranial nerves IX and X are interrupted so that there is difficulty in swallowing and vocalization due to ipsi-

149

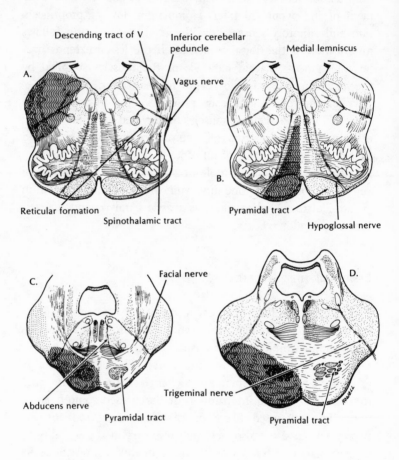

Descending tract of V   Inferior cerebellar peduncle

A.

Medial lemniscus

B.

Vagus nerve

Reticular formation   Spinothalamic tract

Pyramidal tract

Hypoglossal nerve

C.   Facial nerve

D.

Abducens nerve   Pyramidal tract

Trigeminal nerve

Pyramidal tract

38. Lesions of the brain stem

150

lateral palatoplegia and laryngoplegia (paralysis of the vocal cord), respectively. Incoordination of arm and leg movements are evidence of destruction of the inferior cerebellar peduncle (restiform body) and a portion of the cerebellum (hemiasynergia and hemiataxia). Diminished sense of hearing or deafness on the same side may occur on rare occasions if the lesions extend to the cochlear nuclei. There may also be a Horner's syndrome (pupillary constriction, ptosis [drooping eyelid], usually enophthalmus, vasodilatation, and loss of sweat on the same side of the head and face) due to interruption of the descending sympathetic pathways in the reticular formation.

A lesion in the ventromedial medulla (inferior alternating hemiplegia) will usually interrupt the pyramidal tract and exiting fibers of the hypoglossal nerve (Fig. 38B). Involvement of the former results in contralateral hemiplegia (spastic paralysis, exaggerated deep reflexes, positive Babinski). Upon protrusion the tongue will deviate to the side of the lesion due to paralysis of the muscles ipsilateral to the lesion. In time the muscles of the tongue will atrophy. Frequently, the lesion will involve other structures, particularly the dorsally placed medial lemniscus. There will then be a contralateral loss of vibratory and muscle sense.

Middle alternating hemiplegia (Millard-Gubler's syndrome) is usually due to a vascular lesion in the caudal portion of the basal pons (Fig. 38C). Interruption of the exiting fibers of the abducens nerve results in ipsilateral paralysis of lateral gaze due to paralysis of the lateral rectus. There is ipsilateral facial paralysis since the facial nerve is involved. Contralateral hemiplegia, which may include the tongue, is a consequence of interruption of the pyramidal tract.

Another form of alternating hemiplegia results from lesions in the middle pons at the level of the trigeminal nerve (Fig. 38D). The features of this syndrome are ipsilateral paralysis of the muscles of mastication and loss of pain, temperature,

151

and tactile sensibility in the face. There is contralateral hemiplegia, with possible involvement of the tongue, due to interruption of the pyramidal tract.

An acoustic neuroma, which is a tumor of the auditory nerve, will first result in ipsilateral impairment of hearing and signs of vestibular involvement such as nystagmus, vertigo, and tendency to fall to the side of the lesion. (Fig. 39A). As the tumor enlarges it compresses the cerebellar peduncles as evidenced by homolateral asynergy. Another early finding is an absent corneal reflex, indicating trigeminal involvement, probably the descending root. Although the facial nerve accompanies the auditory, its function is rarely impaired. There may be some indication of facial paralysis.

Lesions in the basal portion of the upper pons involve the pyramidal tract and may extend dorsally to the medial lemniscus (Fig. 39B). There is contralateral hemiplegia with positive Babinski and exaggerated deep reflexes. The lower half of the face on the opposite side is also paralyzed. Since the medial lemniscus is also interrupted, muscle and vibratory sense and tactile discrimination are absent contralateral to the lesion.

Persistent coma occurs when the ascending reticular activating system is interrupted bilaterally in the midbrain (Fig. 39C). Usually, the oculomotor nuclei and nerves are also involved, resulting in bilateral ophthalmoplegia characterized by the inability to move the eyes which are fixed forward. There is marked ptosis of both eyelids.

Weber's syndrome (superior alternating hemiplegia) follows lesions in the basis penunculi, which will interrupt the exiting fibers of the oculomotor nerve and pyramidal tract Fig. 39D). There is contralateral hemiplegia with paralysis of the lower half of the face. Homolateral ophthalmoplegia, ptosis of the eyelid, and pupillary dilation are also present.

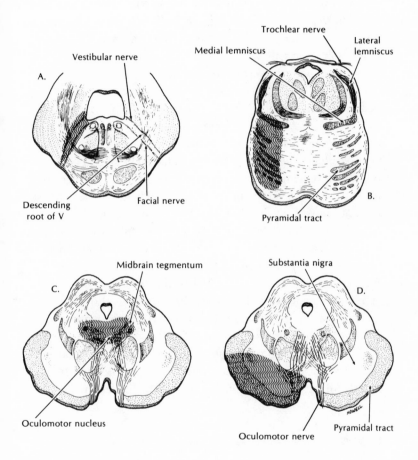

A.

Vestibular nerve

Descending
root of V

Facial nerve

Trochlear nerve

Medial lemniscus

Lateral
lemniscus

Pyramidal tract

B.

C.

Midbrain tegmentum

Oculomotor nucleus

Substantia nigra

D.

Oculomotor nerve

Pyramidal tract

39. Lesions of the brain stem

Lesions of the Cerebellum

In basal and midline cerebellar lesions the patient has difficulty in maintaining an upright position, walks with a wide base, and tends to sway from side to side (Fig. 40). There is no impairment of limb movements and reflexes are normal. Nystagmus may also be present due to the flocculonodular lobe's strong connections with the vestibular system.

Dysfunction resulting from involvement of the cerebellar hemispheres is characterized by hypotonia and ataxia (awkward gait (Fig. 40). All signs indicate a lack of coordination between muscle groups. Therefore, the patient is unable to perform rapidly alternating movements (adiadochokinesis). The direction of movement is inaccurate (past pointing) and there is a tendency to miss the mark (dysmetria). There is a decomposition of movement in that the individual cannot carry out smoothly a complex act such as touching the nose with the finger. A scanning speech may also be evident. The rebound phenomenon can be demonstrated by having the patient flex the forearm against resistance. When this resistance is suddenly removed uncontrolled flexion results. There is also a general weakness of the muscles (asthenia), and the patient tires easily. Nystagmus may also be present. The deep reflexes are diminished and tend to be pendulous. If the lesion involves the deep cerebellar nuclei or brachium conjunctivum an intention tremor occurs. All signs are ipsilateral to the side of the lesion.

Lesions of the Diencephalon

Lesions within the dorsal thalamus result in a condition known as the thalamic syndrome (Fig. 41). The structures involved will determine the signs and symptoms. Thus, there is usually

154

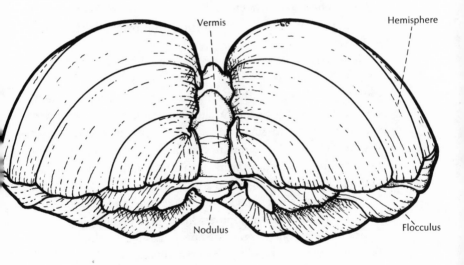

40. Cerebellum (ventral caudal view)

a decrease in pain, and a lessening of temperature and proprioceptive sensations on the side opposite the lesion due to involvement of the ventral posterior nucleus. Impairment of emotional expression, such as unprovoked laughter, is occasionally seen, probably due to involvement of frontothalamic pathways. Atonia and ataxia may occur if the lesion extends anteriorly to the ventral lateral nucleus and termination of the superior cerebellar peduncle. In some patients an intractable pain, which is on the opposite side, may be present. It is usually a severe, generalized burning sensation that may be brought on by the slightest painful or tactile stimulation. It has also been triggered by auditory and visual stimuli. Because of the close proximity of the posterior limb of the internal capsule to the thalamus, the fiber paths within this structure may be interrupted. Thus, a contralateral hemiplegia and/or hemianopsia may be present due to involvement of the pyramidal tract and optic radiations, respectively.

Hypothalamic lesions frequently result in diabetes insipidus (Fig. 41). There is a marked increase in fluid intake and output of urine. It is due either to the interference with production, transport, or storage of the antidiuretic hormone. The structures involved may be the supraoptic nucleus, stalk, or neural lobe of the hypophysis. Other findings in hypothalamic involvement may be impaired temperature regulation, altered food intake, and weight loss or gain. These are due to the role played by the hypothalamus in temperature regulation and metabolism. Through the anterior hypophysis the hypothalamus plays a role in the production of gonadotropins. Lesions within the hypothalamus may, therefore, result in hypogonadism or hypergonadism. Emotion and sleep-wakefulness cycle involve complex neuronal circuitry of which the hypothalamus is a part. Thus, lesions in the hypothalamus, particularly the posterior portion, result in somnolence. Other lesions, which are not well localized, may give rise to irritability, fits of rage, etc.

156

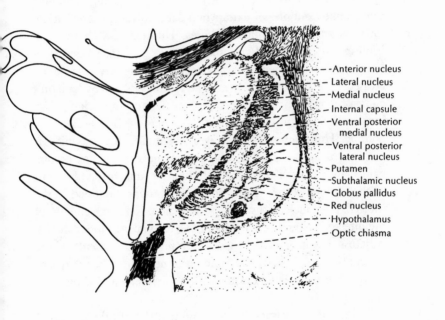

-Anterior nucleus
- Lateral nucleus
-Medial nucleus
- Internal capsule
--Ventral posterior
  medial nucleus
--Ventral posterior
  lateral nucleus
- Putamen
-Subthalamic nucleus
- Globus pallidus
- Red nucleus
- Hypothalamus
-·Optic chiasma

41. Section Through Diencephalon and Basal Ganglia

157

Lesions of the telencephalon

Lesions of the basal ganglia and related extrapyramidal structures are usually diffuse (See Fig. 41). Thus, in any one syndrome of the extrapyramidal system lesions may be found in a wide variety of structures including some outside of this system. The cardinal signs of extrapyramidal disease are the loss of associated movements, which results in a paucity of movement, the presence of an adventitial movement, and an alteration of muscle tone. Some examples of extrapyramidal involvement are Parkinson's syndrome, Sydenham's chorea, Huntington's chorea, ballismus, and athetosis. Parkinson's disease is characterized by a tremor at rest, paucity of movement and rigidity due to increased tone in both the flexors and extensors. In Sydenham's chorea the movements are jerky, irregular, and purposeless. They involve the extremities and face. The muscles ars usually hypotonic. Huntington's chorea is a hereditary disease which is progressive and fatal. The choreiform movements are accompanied by progressive mental deterioration due to involvement of the cerebral cortex. The lesion in ballismus is confined to the subthalamic nucleus, usually on one side. The movements of the affected extremities are spontaneous, violent, and flail-like. Athetosis is characterized by slow, grotesque movements of the extremities, particularly the more distal portions. They may also involve the face. The movements are worm-like and sometimes appear graceful.

Lesions of the primary sensory and motor cortical areas result in deficits referrable to that system (see Fig. 30). Thus, destruction of the precentral gyrus gives rise to contralateral hemiplegia. Involvement of the postcentral gyrus results in contralateral loss of proprioceptive and tactile sensation. When the calcarine cortex is destroyed there is an opposite visual field defect. A patient with a lesion in the prefrontal lobe loses drive, although his intelligence may not be impaired. He is indifferent even to severe pain. There is a release from inhibitions and a lack of responsibility. The individual does not look to the future and is frequently euphoric. However, lesions in the association areas in the parietal, occipital, and temporal lobes, particularly in the dominant hemisphere, do interfere with intellectual processes. Visual agnosia occurs when the lesion is adjacent to the calcarine cortex in the lateral occipital area. The patient is not blind but he cannot recognize, name, or appreciate the significance of an object. Auditory agnosia occurs in posterior temporal lobe lesions. In this case the patient cannot appreciate the spoken word. Proprioceptive and tactile agnosia occurs in posterior parietal lesions. Body parts may not be recognized and objects placed in the hand cannot be identified. Aphasia most often follows lesions in Broca's area in the posterior portion of the inferior frontal gyrus on the dominant side. The patient cannot speak intelligently. He is unable to put words together in a meaningful way. Apraxia, the inability to perform purposive movements, may result from lesions in a wide variety of areas such as the corpus callosum and supramarginal gyrus.

Index

Bouton, 12
Brachium
  of inferior colliculus, 59, 71
  pontis. *See* Peduncle, middle
    cerebellar
  of superior colliculus, 66
Brachium conjunctivum. *See*
    Peduncle, superior cerebellar
Broca's area, 159

Cauda equina, 134
Cell
  epithelial muscle, 1
  hair, 51, 56
  neurosensory, 1
Central acoustic tract, 59, 71
Central canal, 4
Cerebellum, 4
  cortex, layers of, 81
  folia, 80
  vermis, 38, 39, 80
Cerebral aqueduct, 4
Cerebral cortex, 4, 117
Cerebral hemisphere, 4
Cerebrospinal fluid, 127, 133
  composition of, 133
Chorea, 96
  Huntington's, 158
  Sydenham's, 158
Choroid plexus, 16, 133
Chromatolysis, 9, 13
Circle of Willis, 135
Cistern
  interpeduncular, 131
  lumbar, 131, 134
  magna, 131
  pontine, 131
Claustrum, 93
Cochlea, 56
Cochlear duct, 56
Cochlear system, 56
Collateral sprouting, 14
Colliculus
  inferior, 58

superior, 66, 83
Commissure
  anterior, 111, 114
  habenular, 112
  posterior, 67
Communicating ramus, 103
Conductivity, 1
Cordotomy, 32, 50
Corona radiata, 27, 87, 122
Corpora quadrigemina, 4
Corpus callosum, 112
  body, 120
  genu, 120
  rostrum, 120
  splenium, 120
Corpus striatum, 93
Cortex
  association, 27, 38
  auditory, 71, 72, 125
  calcarine, 64
  cerebral, layer of, 117
  entorhinal, 111
  insular, 49, 111, 114, 125
  olfactory, 111
  premotor, 91, 125
  prepyriform, 111
  primary gustatory, 49, 125
  primary motor, 125
  primary sensory, 27, 38, 91,
    122
  septal, 112
  somesthetic, 122
  visual, 122
Crista ampullaris, 51
Cupula, 51

Dendrite, 7, 10
Diabetes insipidus, 108, 156
Diaphragma sellae, 127
Diencephalon, 4
DNA, 7
Dorsal horn, 20
Dorsal root, 7, 20
Dorsal thalamus, 4, 68

167

Transmitters (*Cont.*)
  acetylcholine, 13, 77
  angiotensin, 13
  catecholamine, 13
  dopamine, 13
  endorphin, 13
  enkephalin, 13, 30
  GABA, 13
  glutamic acid, 13
  glycine, 13
  histamine, 13
  neurotensin, 13
  norepinephrine, 13, 99
  serotonin, 13, 30, 99
  substance P, 13, 30
  taurine, 13
Trapezoid body, 58
Tremor, 88
Tricarboxylic acid, 9
Trigeminal neuralgia, 44
Tuber cinereum, 104
Tunnel of Corti, 56

Uncus, 111
Utricle, 51
Uvula, 53, 55

Vein
  anterior spinal, 144
  basilar plexus, 144
  emissary, 141
  great cerebral (of Galen), 141
  inferior cerebral, 141
  inferior ophthalmic, 143
  internal cerebral, 141
  internal jugular, 143
  posterior spinal, 144
  superior cerebral, 141
  superior ophthalmic, 143
Ventricle
  fourth, 5, 133
  lateral, 4, 133
  third, 4, 133
Vertebral venous system, 143
Vertigo, 55